Spikenard

A Woman Anoints Jesus's Feet. Did She Use the Spikenard of Aromatherapy?

Nardostachys jatamansi – An Essential Oil for Digestive Problems, Nervous Disorders, Anxiety, Insomnia, Epilepsy, Seizures and Fear.

-Elizabeth Ashley-

The Secret Healer

To Sherri,
I hope you find this helpful Elizabeth Ashley

1

For Marlys, Anthony, Joshua and Kayla,

a most extraordinary family.

Some things that should not have been forgotten were lost.

History became legend.

Legend became myth

Lord of the Rings - The Fellowship of the Ring

Preface

"... there is one, a bird, which renews itself, and reproduces from itself. The Assyrians call it the Phoenix. It does not live on seeds and herbs, but on drops of incense, and the sap of the cardamom plant. When it has lived for five centuries, it then builds a nest for itself in the topmost branches of a swaying palm tree, using only its beak and talons. As soon as it has lined it with cassia bark, and smooth spikes of nard, cinnamon fragments and yellow myrrh, it settles on top, and ends its life among the perfumes. They say that, from the father's body, a young Phoenix is reborn, destined to live the same number of years. When age has given it strength, and it can carry burdens, it lightens the branches of the tall palm of the heavy nest, and piously carries its own cradle, that was its father's tomb, and, reaching the city of Hyperion, the sun-god, through the clear air, lays it down in front of the sacred doors of Hyperion's temple."

Ovid [1st century CE]

(The Metamorphoses, Book 15, 391-417)

Introduction

This book is about one of the rarest plants on the planet. Its very existence is threatened as it is classed as critically endangered in the wild. It is precious. Its scarcity os not the only reason it is a treasure, for thousands of years it has been one of the most important medicines to the Hindus, and the most incenses to the Brahmen.

A year ago this very weekend, I used it after having experienced the most frightening event of my life. I was amazed at the tranquillity it brought. At Christmas, I wrote about it in a series of blog posts about plants used in the Bible and how it had been used to anoint Christ at Passover, just before his arrest. The historical data I found thrilled me, but some of it seemed to ring untrue. We know there were no "Essential Oils of The Bible" because the process of distillation had not yet been found, but I came across a post saying it had been found in Tutankhamen's tomb, I wondered "How has that passed me by?" With a very keen interest in Egyptology and little bit of knowledge about essential oil, how could I not have known that? Given the extraordinary effects the oil had had on me, earlier in the year, and my fascination for anything smelling vaguely like papyrus, I set off on a quest.

Little, did I know what I was letting myself in for. The world of Spikenard is an absorbing place.

Part of the problem I had was I reluctant to hang the research on a Biblical slant, because whilst many of my readers are staunch Christians, an equal number are not. I was raised in a pagan family, but chose to be confirmed a Christian at 15, partly because the music spoke to my soul so deeply, but partly because I adored the stories from the Bible. Many of you will know that I then went on to study Old Testament archaeology for my A Levels.

Nevertheless, I have come to realise that it is impossible not to use that famous moment of Mary and Jesus at Passover (although there are actually two stories seemingly intertwined perhaps shielding another woman who also anointed the Christ). I feel this way for two reasons:

1. Biblical evidence, Christian and Rabbinic scholars have done the most work in trying to identify the plant source of the oil in the alabaster box.

2. Because ancient *medicinal* texts also refer to Nard, without doing some work into identification of the plant, we would be unable to match what the therapeutic uses were two thousand years ago. Fathoming its Biblical roots – pardon the *Nardostachys*

pun- is essential in understanding how the plant was used.

Luckily for us Ayurvedic medicine was clearer in its recording of history. Unlike Pliny, Galen and Dioscorides they were not cryptic in their recommendations. We know that their medicine was *Nardostachys jatamansi*, the root that you and I now use as the essential oil spikenard.

The story of spikenard is a sensual one. You might recognise its fragrant tones from the erotic Song of Songs, perhaps from tales of the heiro gamos, the sacred union of deity and mortal, or even from the rites of tantra. I'm going to suggest you make this a sensuous journey too. Let fragrance be your guide.

Your experience will be greatly enhanced if you can implement your sense of smell and of sound. I am going to suggest you have your oils box by you as you read. Spikenard of course, you need with you, some others will also serve you well. These are:

- Citronella
- Galangal
- Palmarosa
- Gingergrass

Cinnamon, myrrh and benzoin will also help you to step into some of the most famous moments of history and feel what those people felt all those millennia ago.

Perhaps more than any of the books, music plays a huge part here, because it sets the stage for the reasons the spice was chosen at these events. Its ruling planet is Saturn, the planet of adversity. The sound track I have chosen will help you to see different nuances in the struggles life can bring. If you can find a way to listen to the tracks, I think you will enjoy the book all the more.

Christianity plays a big part between these pages, but so does Judaism, Hinduism and Islam. The medicine is so intrinsically linked with their respective religions it is impossible to detach it, but to my mind that makes the work all the more beautiful. We can see the spirituality of the plant kingdom supersedes the man made divisions and it is a wonder to behold.

Like every plant though, it has its themes; patterns which dictate how its healing might affect the patient. The themes for spikenard seem to go round and round like a carousel, weaving invisible chains of connection between them.

These are:

- Ruling Planet: Saturn

- Archetype: Phoenix
- Emotions: Sacrifice and Great Faith
- Lessons: learning good stuff about yourself, the hard way.

Just for a second you might imagine that you see a flash of gold out of the corner of your eye as the light catches one of these chains.

Possibly

Maybe.

Impossible to know.

And this is most probably the largest of the themes...that you just have to trust your instincts...and know that hope is never far away.

And hope maybe frail...but it is hard to kill.

Come with me on a journey to the beginnings of recorded time. We will honour long forgotten deities and breathe the incense of their majesty.

Discover Biblical texts forgotten through time, such as Christ's circumcision and Moses' vision of Adam and Eve's expulsion from The Garden. If these documents, dating back thousands of years are to be believed then Spikenard played vital parts in both of those events and many, many more.

I hope you have got you sea legs because we will be travelling with The East India Trading Company across to the sunshine and following their work in cataloguing plants and their excitement as they collect wondrous specimens previously seen in the Western world. We'll marvel at their sparkling intellect and comprehensive knowledge of long forgotten languages, and watch as the most magical medicine unfolds and travels across the planet.

History played such a huge part in this book that I have also asked some of my learned aromatic friends if they would like to add their dimensions of how they use the oil to balance it out. Their accounts are spellbinding. Discover how the experts use it in end of life care, to calm terrified animals and even to soothe epilepsy.

The medical world is returning to its roots, quite literally. They are revisiting those ancient wisdoms about this treasured rhizomes and wondering if they can replicate that healing again.

- Could it be true that it can prevent convulsions?
- Make your hair grow darker, fuller and faster…

- Is it possible that it might even be able to heal psychiatric disorders?

We look at the historical arguments, hear the experts opinions and then look over the shoulders of the men in the coats testing the medicine under the microscope.

And then...I promise you we are racing off to buy a bottle!

Spikenard is a medicine than heals any and every troubled souls. It is light in the darkest of times. Ignite that spark and you can kindle something truly amazing to get you through some of the most impossible struggles. Spikenard is the heat that sets that healing alight.

So...are you ready?

Make sure you have your best bib and tucker on. We are about to meet some rather illustrious company. Quietly though, for spikenard is a meditative plant, and we are about to enter hallowed grounds.

Gently does it then.

Let's step inside.

Table of Contents

Part 1: Investigating The Nard of The Ancients

London 1790

Men dressed in finery, with splendid wigs and velvet coats enter a grand white building. From the roof tops, the most exquisite music floats above them. In the past, even the great god Apollo would pause to listen by a well, to the song of the Phoenix. Drowned out by the noise of chatter, the clip clop of the Hansom cab and the thick smog of industrial city, the bird cannot yet be heard.

Yet he watches with interest as these men, whom are so respected and revered, enter Carlton House Terrace, the home of the Royal Society. The bird will strain his feathered ear to listen with interest as to whether these men may finally have discovered what the belovéd "**nard**" of ancient world had been. The leaves of the tree that every ancestor of his line has chosen to build their fragrant nests.

For nigh on five hundred years he has listened with interest and amusement; his father, for five hundred more. So very many eons have passed as the most learned of the humans have wrangled with the identity of the plant, but, thinks the Phoenix, I have nothing if not time.

Inside of the building, members of the Royal Society, the oldest and most prestigious scientific organisation in England, are seated beneath opulently painted ceilings to hear the latest lecture designed to bring a deeper understanding of the natural world. The date is March 18th 1790 and the keynote speaker is a Scottish born physician by the name of Sir Gilbert Blane, a baronet and Physician in Ordinary to the Kings George IV and William IV. The paper he delivers, on this prestigious day, is entitled:

Account of Nardus Indica or Spikenard

He opens with the observation that:

"It is much to be regretted that the records of antiquity afford such imperfect descriptions of natural objects, particularly those of the vegetable kingdom."

He explains how, even though the naturalists of the period, such as Dioscorides and Theophastrus, took great pains to record their *methods* of healing, they would only give the *name* of the plant but rarely gave any botanical description to enable later readers to understand precisely *which* plant they were referring to. Further, observations were usually taken from translations of Latin, Ancient Greek or Egyptian which, ostensibly, are dead languages. So, whilst the plant kingdom is a living breathing entity, that hybridises, evolves and changes, the language we are drawing from does not. Are the plants described in the documents of antiquity even the *same* as those we see today?

The bright purple and gold firebird, smiles to himself impressed by Blane's logic. I wonder, he thought, might this be the man who finally cracks it?

The Phoenix thought it was a good question and so do I. Let's you and I ponder his point for a moment. Are the plants the same? Although years later our generation has high-tech laboratory tests as allies, in many cases for plants like spikenard, or Nard, as we see it referred to in the Bible and other ancient literature, we still cannot say with certainty that we truly understand exactly which plant is being referred to.

Each generation with its scientific and archaeological discoveries has an advantage over the last, of course, and Blane felt he had just such an advantage. His brother had been working in India some years before and had sent him a sample of a grass that Blane felt certain *must be* **The Nard of The Ancients.** He describes a letter from his sibling, dated 1786 from Lucknow (Uttar Pradesh, India).

"Travelling with the Nabob vizier, on one of his hunting excursions, towards the Northern mountains, I was surprised one day, after crossing the river Rapty, about 20 miles from the foot of the hills to perceive the air perfumed with an aromatic smell; and upon walking the cause, I was told it proceeded from the roots of the grass that were bruised or trodden out of the ground by the feet of the elephants and horses of the Nabob's retinue. The country was wild and uncultivated and this was the common grass which covered the surface of it, growing in large tufts close together, very rank, and in general from three to four feet in length. As it was the winter season there was none of it in flower. Indeed the greatest part of it had been burnt down on the road we went, in order that it might be no impediment to the Nabobs encampments. I collected a quantity of the roots to be dried for use and carefully dug up some of it which I sent to be planted in my garden at Lucknow. There it throve exceedingly and in the rainy season it shot up spikes of about 6 ft high. Accompanying this I send you a drawing of the plant in flower and of the dried roots in which the natural appearance, it totally preserved.

It is called by the natives **Terankus** *which means literally in the Hindoo language* **_fever-restrainer_**, *from the virtues they attribute it in that disease. They infuse about a dram of it in half a pint of hot water with a quantity of black pepper. This infusion serves for one dose and is repeated three times a day. It is esteemed a powerful* *medicine in any kinds of fevers whether continued or intermittent. I have not made any trial of it myself but shall certainly take the first opportunity of doing so.*

The whole plant has a strong odour; but both the smell and the virtues reside principally in the husky roots, which in chewing have a bitter warm taste accompanied with the same degree of a kind of glow in the mouth that cardamoms occasion."

So, armed with the drawing and the description, the plant was given, by Blane, to Sir Joseph Banks of the Royal Society, and he was able to identify this plant as being from the species *Andropogon*. (The talented botanists amongst you will connect that to Lemongrass and actually Vetiver too, since that is sometimes written *Andropogon zizanoides*. As it is, Blane is speaking as a plant *Andropogon nardus*, the modern day synonym is *Cymbopogon nardus* which is what you and I know as Citronella.) This was very different from any other plant that had been previously suspected to have been the Nard of the Ancients. (And I'll explain why that is in a moment.)

The Phoenix was fascinated. This fellow, Blane, was indeed a charismatic orator and he was transfixed by the Scotsman's theories. What the bird wanted to know was: what was it about this letter that had inspired Blane to suspect that he

may have uncovered the identity of the enigmatic plant that *everyone* wanted to name?

Well, Blane remembered a passage he had read by the Roman commentator Arrian had, in the First Century, quoted from an earlier writer Aristobulus and spoken of Alexander The Great's passage into India. Here, Arrian had reported that the army marched through the deserts of Gadriosia, a maritime province of Persia, situated between Kerman and the river Indus; it being the frontier of Persia towards India. He described how the air was perfumed by the spikenard that the army trampled underfoot, and how Phoenicians accompanying the expedition collected large quantities to carry to their own country to sell. The Phoenicians were legendary for their commercial prowess and it was understood that if they were interested in a commodity, then you could be assured that it had a high worth. (You might remember from my blogs about plants in The Bible how they had become incredibly affluent because they had control of the wood from the Cedars of Lebanon.)

I can see what Blane means. This trampling does certainly sound to be the same experience, doesn't it?

He, then, describes how he has compared details he has found in other classical texts, about this Nard of the Ancients and asserts that the plant must be from the genus *graminicae* because in other ancient documents he has found it referred to as *arista*. Arista was appropriate naming for *grasses* and *grains*, which the Ancient Greeks particularly used to denote the edible parts of plants, like seeds, that they deemed beneficial for animal fodder.

Then he goes on to regale different etymology behind the word **Spikenard**. *Spica* referring to plants which are *verticillatae*. These have spike-like and very fragrant blossoms. He reminds his eminent Royal Society guests that the Romans referred to lavender as *Nardus Italica*, but describes how he has never come across a mention of this Nardus italica also being arista (i.e. he never saw lavender listed as grass for animals to eat) and so concludes these *Nardus italica* and *Nardus indica* must be separate and different things. Nardus indica must stand alone as something entirely unique.

I mentioned earlier that there had long been controversy over its identification and that Blane's Andropogon suggestion was extremely original. This is because even the writers of antiquity would separate this Nard into many, many different varieties, but as time went by, it became ever more unclear as to whether these Nardin (just one of the plurals you will come across for Nard!) that the ancients had so beloved, were even belonging to the same plant family at all.

Both the poets and naturalists of antiquity gave a weighted, almost reverent specialism to *Nardus indica,* clearly elevating this to a superior standard calling it **True Nardus.** Statius (a Roman poet from 1st Century AD) calls it *odoratae aristae.*(Here's Blane's horse food comment again, you notice?) Then, Blane relates how Ovid, exiled for his uninhibited verse, describes spikenard as one of the materials used to create the Phoenix nest and calls it **Nardi levis aristmatic.** The bird, which lived to be 500 years old (or Pliny says 660yrs) did not eat fruits or flowers, but instead feasted on Frankincense and odorous gums. As the bird senses death approaching, it builds itself a nest, a funeral pyre made of many aromatic objects. A poem ascribed to Lactantius (an early Christian author from c250-350 AD, who was to later become adviser to Constantine I) describes these objects in more detail than Ovid has, Again he mentions spikenard, but also cinnamon, amomum, cassia and acanthus. He says *his addit teranus Nardi pubentis aristas,* which translates roughly to "to this he adds the juicy corn Nardi" so yet again we see this *aristas* that Blane was so interested in, and he is right, there does seem to be an idea of animals feed or at least bedding here, doesn't there? In addition to this, the word *"pubentis"* is the name that is used in Linnaean plant classification to signify other plants which we now recognise to be from the Andropogon genus.

Theophastrus, in the 3rd Century BC, was probably the first Greek to mention Nard. He claims it to be a root, from India and has a biting hot taste and resembles the iris root in that it perfumes the air locally. He tells us "The best comes from India" and that it is the most durable of perfumes.

Pliny agrees, saying the "Sincere Nard" is known by its reddish colour, sweet smell and especially its taste "For it drieth the tongue and leaveth a pleasant relish behind it." He is a tad confusing though because, he tells us that both spike and leaf are in use. What does that mean? Spike flowers or the spikey lower leaves? Impossible to know.

You'll remember one of my favourite sources Galen? The Roman doctor who first understood that illness was something that came from within, rather than being some kind of affliction from the gods? His writings may clarify things a little or make things more confusing, depending on which way you look at it, because he is explicit in his instruction that **there are many different types of Nardu.** He is clear, however, that **Nardus indica is the only one which should be referred to as spikenard**. He also speaks of *Nardus* *celtica*, which is now generally accepted to be a plant of the valerian family. Theophastrus tells us "Most fragrant of aromatics come from Asia, while from Europe comes nothing but the iris" suggesting that this celtic nard was more than just a little inferior to the Indian.

Now, we find our first fly in Blane's ointment (and you will come to see that there are many!) He accepts that the sample he has given to Banks in no way resembles the *Nardus Indica* described by Pliny. Pliny had described the specimen used in *his* healing as *"frutex radice pingui et crassâ"*, and that translates to *a fat root and plant.* So the <u>small </u>fibrous roots Blane held in *his* hand had, he admitted, given him pause. He felt though that this could be explained because his sample had come directly to him from India and since Italy was a long way from the plant's origin, and given Nard's high value, perhaps Pliny had procured some lesser substitute from a dodgy dealer and not been able to tell the difference.

Usefully to us, he cites some other sources of ancient references to this ancient Nard to add weight to his argument. He recounted how the First Century Roman poet Horace had included *Nardus Assyria* in his tales. He detailed how Dioscorides, like Galen had been clear that *Nardus Syriaca* was a very different species from *Indica*, but that actually both

28

sources had taken great pains to explain that sometimes **True Nard would be known as Nardus Gangites**....or as being collected from the mountains near where the Ganges flows, and as having a blackish root, with short spikes and smelling something like cypress. He also tells us that *Syriaca* was not named after Syria, but that it grew in the mountains that ran from India to Syria. The Syrian Nard, he said had a fragrance not dissimilar to galangal. "It is spicy and dries the tongue and leaves an agreeable odour in the mouth if chewed for a long time.

In his work though, Pliny lists 12 different types of Nard in Natural History, some have been identifiable as *Lavender stoechas*, *Polianthes tuberose*, *Valeria officinalis* and the True Nard that we are concerned with. He also tells us that since Nardus Indica was hard to get, the Romans began replacing with a herb *Saliunca*, this is widely accepted to be *Nardus celtica* or *valeria offinalis* L. Pliny tells us it was found in the Alps and Balkan regions and because it was of such wonderful quality, it became a veritable gold mine for region.

As to the Indian Nard, there is a surprise, because Galen says it is of *inferior* quality because of the humidity of the area of its origin. He relates that the spikes are longer and it has a larger spike, and the fibres are more intermingled. "Its odour is noxious. The Nard which comes from the *interior of the mountain* is superior to the other, having a shorter spike and having the fragrance of galangal and otherwise resembling the Syrian."

Now, like I say, Blane's argument did seem very convincing, albeit with the odd mosquito in the unguentum but the people in the know *seemed* to be happy with what he had said.

Amongst those pondering Blane's theories, was Sir Joseph Banks, the man who had identified the specimen for him. Banks was a brilliant naturalist and botanist who had amongst other things accompanied Captain James Cook on his voyages to New Zealand and Australia. On his return, his recording of new plants had brought him instant recognition. He consulted at Kew Gardens for the King and was really responsible for the extraordinary collection of specimens it has today. He despatched botanists all over the world and kept a keen line of communications with other ambassadors abroad asking about gaining specimens for Kew Gardens to study.

As heads were nodding, convinced by Blane's arguments, another man by the name of Sir William Jones was working in India, but he seemed far from happy with Blane's thoughts.

In a correspondence, Sir William Jones wrote to Sir Joseph Banks on October 18th 1791. He begins:

I thank you heartily for your kind letters, but perhaps I cannot express my thanks better than by answering them as exactly I am able.

First as to sending plants from India, I beg you to accept my excuses, and make them to George Young, for my apparent inattention to such commissions. In short if you wish to transfer our Indian plants to the Western islands, the Company must direct Kyd and Roxburgh to send them, and to attend to them". Sir William continues to describe how shorthanded they are without a botanist because theirs is suffering from headaches. Then the letter turns to what must have been a reference to Sir Joseph asking Jones what *he* thought about Blane's ideas at the lecture, and Sir William says....

*"As to Nard, I do not know what to say. If the Greeks meant only fragrant grass then we have nards in abundance, acorusm, schoenusm, andropogon, cyperus etc. But I have no evidence that they meant any such thing. On Arrian, or rather Aristobulus we cannot safely rely as they place cinnamon in Arabia and Myrrh in Persia. Should any travelling botanist find the species of Andropogon, mentioned by Mr Blane in the plains of Gedrosia, it **would** be some evidence, but would at the same time prove that it*

31

*was **not** the Indian nard, which was never supposed to grow in Persia. As at present I believe the Indian nard of the ancients to have been a valerian, at least the nard of Ptolemy, which brought from the very country mentioned by him as famed for the spikenard."*

(It will serve you well to get a translation of some of his grasses mentioned here. Schoenusm is *Andropogon schoenanthus* - also known as *camels hair* or *lemongrass*. *Acorus calamus* is a grass known as *sweet flag*. Cyperus is a large genus of triangular leafed sedges.)

As it is, Sir William Jones, is nearing the end of his life when he writes this letter, but the last four years until his sad demise become entirely fascinated by Jones's own search for the True Nardus. Before his death he wrote a paper which was to become vitally important in the search for identification of the plant. His 1790 treatise opens with words which seem to echo my oft thought notions about my own work and so I instantly felt a deep kinship with the man. He says:

"This is intended as an apology for the pains which have been taken to procure a determinate answer to a question that seems to have no apparent utility...."

Yes, entirely useless question, I wholeheartedly agree, Sir William. But nevertheless, I am eager to know your thoughts.

"[a question] that should best be answered in India....What is Spikenard?""

To search in India, for an answer, seems to be logical to me. Pray tell us more, kind Sir.

Jones had amassed astounding amounts of evidence from classical literature. Not least he had discovered that the Egyptian physician Ptolemy (AD100-170), whom he spoke of, had given a description of his spikenard growing on the borders of Rangamritica and Rangamati which is what we would now know as Bhutan, which was very close to where Jones was living in India. So he set off on a wondrous voyage of discovery, immersing himself in the land and culture of the region to see if he could learn, amongst other things, the identity of True Spikenard.

During my research, I came across completely unrelated letter Jones had sent to a friend which I think adds a lovely context to how he had managed to come to his conclusions about what Nardus indica might be. On Sept 27th 1787, he wrote to Thomas Caldicott esq

"Your brother sent me you[r] letter at a convenient time and to a convenient place, for I can only write in the long vacation, which I generally spend in a delightful cottage, about as far from Calcutta as

Oxford is from London, and close to an ancient university of Brahmans with whom I now converse familiarly in Sanscrit. You would be astonished at the resemblance between that language and both Greek and Latin. Sanscrit and Arabic will enable me to do this country more essential service than the introduction of the arts (even if I should be able the introduce them) by procuring an accurate digest of the Hindu and Mohammeden laws, which the natives hold sacred, and by which both justice and policy require that they should be governed.

I have published nothing; but the Armenian clerks make such blunders that I print ten or twenty copies of everything I compose, which are to be considered manuscripts. I beg you will send me your comments on these"

(I couldn't help but wonder if he would love or totally distrust email, when I read this!)

In his treatise later, he illustrates how his largest problems in getting any identification on what Nard might be, was as ever with knowing what name he should be using – the ultimate Catch 22.

Nard, he explained had been classified by Hebrew lexicographers labouring under a misapprehension. They had presumed that the exotic Nard was an Indian word, but instead he had found it to be Persian. That instead of being the name of a *plant,* Nard had been taken by the Arabs from the name from the aforementioned unguent or ointment as was used to anoint Christ, and as such historians were trying to locate a plant using a name of a lotion or perfume!

The Persian or Arabic name for spike or ear, however, is also seen in the translation to Sumbul, which is the local's name for their medicinal plant....Nardostachys.

He explained that a doctor from Delhi had argued that the plant was not jatamansi, but Sâd as they know it in Arabic. The doctor had then shown him an entry in the Persian Dictionary of Natural History which had the following translation.

1. Sâd has a roundish olive shaped root, externally black, but white internally, and so fragrant as to have obtained in Persia the name of Subterranean Musk; its leaf has some resemblance to that of a leek, but is longer and narrower, strong, somewhat rough at the edges and tapering to a point.

2. Sumbul means "a spike or ear" **and was called Nard by the Greeks.** There are three types of Sumbul or Nardin; but when the word stands alone it means Sumbul of India, which is a herb without fruit or flower, like the tail of an ermine, or of a small weasel, but not quite so

thick, and about the length of a finger. It is darkish inclining to yellow and very fragrant it is brought from Hindustan and its medical virtue lasts three years"

When later Sir William spoke to priests and Brahmen at the university they described how they added the Sumbul into their sacrifices. They told him that when it was fresh it smelled incredibly sweet and so was added in large quantities to scent rich essence and perfumes. Merchants would venture to the mountainous country just north east of Bengal to buy it, they said. There though, Jones regales, they would buy the whole plant and not only the roots. Thus it had gained a Sanscrit name from the resemblance the shaggy hairs on the lower stems – which is the part that holds the perfume - had to locks of hair. Jones, like Blane too, wonders at the distance between the origins of the plant and the ancient destination of the journey, but this time says that since the Ancient Greeks could never have seen the plant in bloom, and thus not understood the "Spikes". He could see how the name SpikeNard might have never quite worked, and instead the famous perfume became its name.

Several times through his paper he refers to how the author of *Tohfatul Momineen*, a late 18th Century Unani pharmacopeia describes the Sumbul of India as the "Sweet Sumbul" but that he had described it as a denomination of the same sumbul specimen that his physician had brought to him...that of jatamansi.

What is important to understand here is Jones was never able to gain the opportunity of seeing a live plant. All of his work had been based on dried specimens and comparisons with a drawing by an East India surgeon, Adam Burt. This will become important later, when we look at the botany. For now though, let's move on.

So, at the turn of the century, Sirs Blane and Jones had brought us a little closer to understanding what this Nard used in the Bible and other great events in the Ancient world might have been. Spikenard was almost certainly, as Linneaus had categorised it, some kind of grass and most possibly was Nardostachys jatamansi. But from that first reading of the paper by Blane to the Royal Society and then a small counter offer by Jones, little else was brought to the *historical* table of learning until a member of the Pharmaceutical Society of St Petersburgh and Academie Royal des Sciences, Charles Hatchett published "On The Spikenard of the Ancients" in 1836. It was Hatchett's turn to play *his* advantage.

Six years before, a friend had visited him after having spent 34 years in India, in Malvah, and with him Samuel Swinton esq had brought some Oil of Spikenard. It is the first bottle of spikenard to ever come to England.

Swinton, it seems, had been in the employ of The East India Company and had been severely afflicted with rheumatism. After many years of suffering, the natives had suggested he try what they called *Rhonsee Ke Teel*, which means **Oil of Grass.** He complied and was so excited by how well it had worked, had sent it to his cousin, George Swinton, who was a government official. He, in turn had been impressed and so had given it to a Dr William Russell (later to become Sir) and a colleague of Russell's, to test its virtues further. (Spikenard really is the tale of the Old Boy's network, isn't it? Every one of them has been knighted and landed up in the House of Lords!)

Satisfied and also having taken note of comments from the natives, they agreed that the oil seemed to be superb for rheumatism. But what they also found was even more remarkable, that no-one seemed to know of the oil outside of the immediate vicinity of where it grew; The Old Boys could not tell if that was accidental or if the plant had been deliberately kept secret from the government. Either way despite how wonderfully the medicine worked, until Swinton had communicated with his cousin, its favours had remained entirely under the radar. Now, Hatchett then places another buzzing beastie in our Nardus ungenteum because he explains that he showed Swinton the engraved plate which accompanied *Blane's* paper, of the Andropogon, that Swinton agreed that *it* was the correct plant. Further, whilst the plant did grow in other parts of India, as well as in Malvah, it was those grown around the Jaum Ghaut that were the most revered. He detailed how the plants were gathered in October, when the seed-forming ears or spikes were fully formed. When the rains came, the grass would grow enormous and jungle fever was rife so unless the most hungry of peasants had been tempted with the promise of very high pay, no-one would venture up to harvest it. This of course would explain the incredibly high price that the oil/ ointment could demand, and also that it could only possibly be afforded by the very top castes of the natives.

Apparently the oil had been prepared in Malvah "since time immemorial" at first by the parsee, but then at the time of Swinton's residence by the Borahs, an extremely commercial tribe who formed a Muslim sect in the area. The oil, he described was formed from the ripe spikes with a foot long section of stem, then this was taken for *distillation*. If this is true, and there is no reason to doubt that it is, even if the oil may possibly not have been the Nard of the Ancients...well, that would mean that the Arabs were not the first to discover distillation...it had been happening secretly in these hills for eons before.

Just the smallest quantity of the liquid was used by the natives, at the time of Hatchett's writing, just as it had been two thousand years before. The remainder of the oil, according to local lore, was sent to Tarsus to be sold as an ingredient for the celebrated ointment. This ointment was described as thin but deliciously fragrant liquid, with spikenard (whatever that plant maybe- Andropogon in this tale) as the principal ingredient, but would have been blended with costus orientalis, Myrrh or Balsam of Gilead.

Local legend said that the ointment was only really prepared in Tarsus and Laodicea with the process being kept secret to only the most sacred few. (It's like Kentucky Fried chicken, isn't it?). Swinton illustrated that the price was so high that it would always be kept in special boxes. Small amounts were given in Onyx or agate, and larger ones in alabaster. And, at the end of the 1st Century AD, perfume writer Apollonius the Heriphilon, writes, in his treatise *"On Perfumes* "that essence of Spikenard is the best from Tarsus."

Pliny wrote that one should sprinkle one's clothes with Nard to make them smell bright. Maybe the olfactory trands have changed a great deal over two thousand years but I can't imagine wanting to stink of spikenard or valerian all day, and I would not describe either as being "bright". Gingergrass, by contrast, yes that would be more likely to work for me.

It is worth pausing here and recognising that Blane in particular was probably not aware that any such thing as an Oil of Spikenard existed because he had originally commented thus:

"It may here be remarked that its sensible qualities do not depend on a principle so volatile as essential oil like most other aromatic vegetables, this would be a great recommendation to the ancients, as its virtues would be more durable, and they were not acquainted with the method of collecting essential oils being ignorant of the art of distillation". Strangely, possibly they may *not* have been ignorant of distillation if Hatchett's assertion had been correct, that Blane had been accurate that Nard *was* Andropogon and that it had been distilled "since time immemorial".

So, let's take a moment to look up at the Phoenix soaring above us. Hear its beautiful song as he collects all the knowledge and wisdom of this age. And, just for a second, decide whose argument has swayed us the most. As the 19th century opens it brings with it one of spikenard's busiest times in history. It is a time when it has done most good.

41

As Hatchett writes, little does he know that the plant that Jones had described, not the Andropogon, but the jatamansi was becoming a healing superstar on the other side of the planet.

Across the world, a disease is spreading at a terrifying rate. A disease, it was supposed was spread by contact with filth and decay. Cholera was killing thousands of people a week in Europe and the USA. Physicians and lay people alike suspected that debauched lifestyles were to blame. Sermons were preached in churches and riots broke out as mass burials tried to deal with the growing problem of the dead.

It seems to be a strange disease, this cholera. Paradoxical somehow, because as the death toll rises at an alarming rate, the fact that physicians attending to the afflicted seem to remain well, leads to the conclusion that it cannot be contagious. It will be another 20 years in 1855 when John Snow will identify that drinking contaminated water is the problem and another 18 years after that, until Robert Koch finally identifies the *cholera bacillus*. But still, people struggle to understand the ramifications of this in terms of is it/isn't it contagious?

And so it continued that people would drink contaminated water, would develop unbelievable diarrhoea and become so speedily dehydrated that their blood would thicken, their eyes would become sunken into their heads and their skin would turn blue. The diarrhoea would become like a straw coloured liquid that would almost invisibly soak the sheets. Carers would change the beds unaware of the importance of washing their hands, and then, of course, proceed to prepare food.

Between 1832 -1866, Britain suffered four cholera epidemics, each more terrible than the one before. Spreading from its source in the Ganges, it travelled across Europe, to Britain and even as far as America and Australia.

The context for the disease in England was a strange one and societal changes of the period fuelled the danger that the illness brought. A new bill had recently been passed through the House of Commons for Parliamentary reform, most relevantly giving the ordinary man the right to vote. The country wanted change after becoming disenchanted by the overly indulgent ways of George IV. Britain had had enough of misappropriation of power at the top. These political changes meant that not only wealthy landowners could also have a route to power, but blue collar workers too. Understandably the aristocracy were appalled at the notion and they over turned the bill in the House of Lords.

Many people suspected that stories of cholera were simply political spin to divert attention away from the reform bill. Many even suggested that cholera did not even exist. The Lords debated and dithered for months and the mood of the country grew tense. Like a melting pot the pressure exploded into riots across the country.

These changes were very important to the Black Country where I am from, because in the midst of the Industrial Revolution hundreds of people gravitated to these thriving towns in a bid to find engineering work. When the reform bill was passed in June 1832, it meant that one in six adult men could vote and although the electorate only raised a small amount from 400,000 – 650,000, there was a shift in the kind of people involved. Suddenly it's not just your Lord Granthams who can wield power but people from manufacturing and commerce too. Consequently these towns, which had grew with terrifying speed, suffered terrible losses of human life from cholera.

In Bilston, part of Wolverhampton where I grew up, 700 people were lost in two months. The same houses still stand in the area. Red brick terraces, all built one on top of the other. There is no way the sanitation in the area would have been able to cope with the economic boom. By 1841 the population in Bilston was counted at 20,180 people, having more than trebled since 1801 when the figure stood at just 6,914. Thousands of people, all following the smoke to the factories smelting iron and leading the whole world in engineering, unbeknownst to them, were heading to their deaths. Thirty seven of that 700 lived in one small street, Temple Street.

So as this new political environment changes, everyone is speculating as to the *cause* of the cholera, where does it come from. Does it even exist? The panic is made worse by another parliamentary bill that is passed in '32 to furnish the universities and hospitals with a means to research this and other diseases. Government stipulates that anybody not claimed by the family for burial within 48 hours can be offered up for dissection, in a bid to prevent the grave robbing that has become so problematic.

So as people become sicker, they are shipped off to special cholera hospitals and can die in as little as 24 hours. Many families are terrified that their loved ones are being *killed* to fuel the government's cholera "stories." In response they would picket the hospital and often spark off terrible riots. Minutes from one particular hospital meeting recorded: *"The bodies of those who have died have been removed as speedily as possible, but in the case of the young woman who died in Vine*

Street, about 200 and [sic] 300 persons collected to prevent the removal of the body. It was, therefore, not persisted in"

The church in its eminent wisdom suspected that this must be divine vengeance for avarice and vice and ordered a national day of fasting. The media went wild and papers were full of satirical cartoons suggesting that perhaps the poor had fasted enough. Incited again...the hoards took to the streets and found another cause about which to riot.

I feel it is important to understand the political context to comprehend how the next part of our story could possibly have been overlooked. Over the smog of the revolution, the screams of writhing abdominal pain and the anger and grief of the masses, it must have been impossible to hear the Phoenix song as she carried her fragrant branches above.

In fact, the bird was not the only one trying to make people hear.

In 1850 The Edinburgh Medical and Science Journal published *A Concise View of The Latest and Most Important Discoveries in Medicine, Surgery and Pharmacy*, and contained therein was a chapter written by a certain Dr A. B. Granville.

It is entitled:

The Sumbul: A new Asiatic remedy of great power against nervous disorders, spasms of the stomach, cramp, hysterical affections, paralysis of the limbs, and epilepsy: with an account of its physical, chemical and medicinal characters and a specific property of checking the progress of collapse cholera as first ascertained in Russia.

Snappy headline, don't you think?

Augustus Bozzi Granville was a naturalised British physician who had been born in Milan in 1783. He had originally studied medicine as a means to avoid military training under Napoleon. After graduating medical college, he practiced in Greece, Turkey, Spain and Portugal. Then, Granville joined the British Navy. Travelling extensively, he learned to speak and write English both fluently and eloquently.

Granville is especially remembered for his work in cholera *prevention*, as well as having been the first physician to do a post mortem on an Egyptian mummy. He also introduced several new ingredients into the British materia medica. These included prussic acid (a horrible poison that has since been used to make chemical weapons and to kill Jews in Aushwitz) and the *Sumbul* – that is *Nardostachys jatamansi*, or as aromatherapists of today refer to it, spikenard.

He had been first introduced to the practice of using sumbul when he had been invited to St Petersburg to observe how the Russian doctors were treating cholera.

In that published article, we get a sense of man who is frustrated, angry and quite incensed. I am not convinced that he would be the first person to be bewildered by the English medical authorities. He relates how he has published papers about how The Sumbul was treating and saving hundreds of lives from cholera in Russia. The articles had run in The Times and four other English journals, all of which he assures the reader, were favourably commented upon, especially in the Pharmaceutical Journal of London and the English Gazette. Nevertheless he can see no evidence of anyone trying to emulate its usage in England.

Within 2 years of usage in Russia, Sumbul had gained considerable fame for its affects on the worst stages of cholera. Previously it had been used a stimulant or tonic for livestock with advanced stages of malignant fevers or with dysentery and chronic diarrhoea. The drug had shown unquestionable success.

The physicians of Moscow were in the closest proximity of the herb when cholera had first broken out and had been able to procure it swiftly and easily, then had used it to the greatest effect. He relates:*"They hesitate not to ascribe its virtues in the saving of thousands of lives in the latest epidemic."*

He tells us that, by contrast, the English daily death toll rose from 823 on Aug 11th 1847 to 2026 (each day) by the 12th of September, but yet he can see no evidence of anyone having carried out any of the recommendations in the papers he had written to such wide medical acclaim. Poor Granville. He must have been utterly bewildered as to why his exciting news of a cure had been entirely overlooked. However in retrospect, it is easier for *us* to see how that might have been.

Dr Granville was not to be discouraged and he was eager to understand why no one had taken up his advice. His research revealed that one of the reasons was that, rather than being a usual ingredient that people would be aware of, none of the apothecaries he had showed the sunbul to seemed to recognise it. He had searched English materia medica but had only managed to find one solitary entry by a Dr Periera, written in the Pharmaceutical Journal, very recently, in 1848. Periera reports how he found *his* drug in St Petersburg, and that he also knew that Dr Martiny of Dharmstadt had employed it with success in treating dropsies. (Dropsy = Oedema to me, edema or swelling to most of you!)

He then speaks of a colleague Mr Savory who had gone to great lengths to procure some of the drug, but had been so far, unsuccessful.

When finally Mr. Savory had had the chance to have a taste and sniff of the root that Granville had, he concluded that the fragrance was so powerful, that it must have incredibly potent properties too. Finally, after much time and great expense Savory had been able to gain enough of a sample of the drug to be able to make a tincture from it, and he suspected that it might be a very useful treatment to use on patients with epilepsy after he had read an analogy of a herb called "Musk" being written in the Lancet in 1850.

Granville, by now had been collecting jatamansi for about 9 years. The Bootan agents that had that he had originally procured it from had stated that it was principally for the bowels, but he had been very busy making his own tinctures, decoctions, alcoholic and ether extractions as well as powders for his own therapeutic experimentations. He started to use them on patients with "Disordered nerves and such as the details in the title". (And written in that context we can see that the overly restrictive controls we now have from the Medicines Controls Board and the FDA might not be *such* a bad thing!)

He describes how he had found a selection of these roots when he had visited a warehouse in Heidelberg, Germany. The manager related how they had been there a very long time but that sadly, when they had been used to try to treat the epidemic when it had broken out in Mannheim, the effects were completely inert. The druggist had tried to apply for more of it from St Petersburg, so as to have a newer and perhaps more efficacious sample but he was told that there had been so much of the root used in the epidemic that it would be very difficult to procure any more until there had been fresh imports.

But the question then was...

Import from where?

Granville says:

"It is a mistake to suppose it grows in Hindustan. At least under the time of Sir William Jones, it was not found in any part of India under the sway of the British. It appears it is a native of Bhootan and the mountains of Nepal" Then he offers *" considerable amounts of jatamansi (that is the dried plant) is brought in by caravans, but by law living plants cannot be exported without a license from the sovereign".*

Actually, it seems that there are many suggestions from experts: Constantinople, Trebisand, Nidjin, Norgorod are all offered as possibilities. Botanists Ermann and Von Ledebour however have told Granville that they feel the plant's habitat must be: *"Bucharia, a district to the north of Mount Thibet and part of the Mongol Empire"*

But, he says, the dealers of Sunbul, *they* say it comes from Persia.

Then he directs his reader to Dr Royle's *"Illustrations of Botany From The Himalayan Mountains"*. J. Forbes Royle had said in 1839, "Sunbul, pronounced Sumbul, designates three of four different vegetable products."

Can you hear the Phoenix above? He is positively wetting himself, screeching in laughter at us.....*Three or four more possibilities* !!!!

Dr Royle said he was in agreement with William Jones.

Or at least he had been...until he had been shown a plant. Now you will recall that Jones had never been able to secure a live specimen of the plant to compare, so he was at a disadvantage to Royle who seems, despite this export embargo on live plants, had managed to get to see one.

He reminds us that Jones's translations about Sumbul from Persian dictionaries had said:

"The hyacinth – The spikenard to which the mistresses hair is compared. Ears of Corn. That it was considered synonymous with the Nardos of the Ancient Greeks."

But, says Royle, on consulting *Mukhsun ool Udrich* and other Persian works he had found in India, the plant had been shown as "Narden" in the Index, but then had been always referred to as Sumbul in the body text. In other words there seemed to be several sumbul that made up the Narden classification.

More, it had been sub classified into four types of sumbul.

- *Sumbul lindee*
- *Sumbul-roomee* or *ukletee* which was sometimes also called *narden ukletee.*
- *Sumbul jibulee* or *mountain nard*
- *Sumbul farsee*

Narden ukletee, he surmised must have been the specimen that Dioscorides had spoken of called *Sumbul italioon* – that is Nard that grows in Italy (And that Blane had asserted was lavender, if you are struggling to keep up!)

Also he tells us that *Polianthes tuberose* is also described as being one of the kinds of Persian sunbul. Tuberose? TUBEROSE...Pliny said that too, didn't he? That means there are the three different types of Sumbul which might be Nard, but at least we are happy that it is one certain type of Nardostachys jatamansi.

He also takes Hatchetts' Andropogon assumption to task and fills in some blanks for us. He tells us that many people erroneously ascribe the Oil of Grass to *Andropogon Ivrandcusa*, *but he knows it to come from Andropogus Calamus aromaticus*, and that that the Grass Oil of Namur, might also have been "the sweet cane" and the "rich aromatic reed from a far country" of scripture. That this Grass Oil is extensively used in India for the external application in rheumatism, the same way as cajeputi is also used and that it was also given as a stimulant.

Andropogus Calamus aromaticus is the plant that has been later classified as *Cymbopogon Martinii....Gingergrass or palmarosa*. I whole heartedly agree gingergrass is a wonderful treatment for rheumatism. But is it Nard? I'm so dizzy I have no idea! Let's carry on our search... Nardostachys jatamansi

Identification and Taxonomy

Experts now accept that Jones was correct that the Sunbul was the Indian Nard of Antiquity. It seems likely that Andropogon was used as another of the Nards. For a moment, though I want to take your mind back to our notes on William Jones's assertions about Nardostachys, because we are still not home and dry.

There was one real problem with his treatise. Unbeknownst to him, he had accidentally obtained two parts of two different plants. The roots and the ariel parts of the plants did not match. The roots were correct but the ariel parts of the plants were later identified as coming from yet another member of the Valeriana genus, *Valeriana hardickii.*

Then in 1795, Dr Roxburgh (remember him from letters to Banks?) inadvertently further added to the confusion when he published a specimen based on Jones's notes and named it Valeriana Jatamansi. William Roxbugh is known as the Founding Father of Indian Botany. He employed dozens of Indian artists documenting native plant specimens. By 1790, he already had 700 illustrations. He was later asked to fill the position of superintendant of Calcutta Gardens when Colonel Robert Kyd (also mentioned in Jones's letters) had died.

Roxburgh sent many illustrations to Joseph Banks. He began publishing in May 1795 "Plants for the Coromandel" in three volumes which comprised 300 drawings and descriptions. The final part was published in 1820. His journal, later to cause the confusion reads:

November 6th 1794

I received from the honourable C. A Bruce, commissioner at Coos Beyhar, two small baskets with plants of this valuable drug. He writes to me in 27th September (so long had the plants been on the road) that he had, the day before, received them from the Deb Rajan of Bootan; and further says that the Booteans know the plant by two names, viz Jatamansi and Pampé or Paumpé.

Now the story takes an unexpected but satisfying turn by way of a young man by the name of David Don, a Scottish botanist, who was later to become professor of Botany at Kings College London and a librarian of the Linnaean society. Don was a bright shining star, classifying many conifers and in 1836 established the new orchid genus *Pleinone*. He had looked at Jones and Roxburgh's notes and shook his head. He could see the error and tried to remedy the situation by applying the binomial "True Jatamansi". The problem was that he saw the error but jumped on the wrong piece of information to rectify it. Rather than focusing on Jones's description, or even

Roxburgh's plate, he zeroed on a note Jones had made about a conversation a friend of his "Harrington" had had with two traders from Bhutan.

In 1825, Don then stepped back and changed his mind. He announced that Valeriana was not the true jatamansi after all and so renamed it yet again as Patrina jatamansi.

This was a completely new species as far as classification was concerned. Back in '21 Don had been a bit cagey about where he had obtained the specimen from citing it as "Bootiniae and Nepaliene Alpibus" but in 25 he was more forthcoming citing his source as a collector by the name of "Wallich".

Nathaniel Wallich was a Danish botanist appointed to be assistant to Roxburgh as East India Company's botanist. After having found an interest in flora, he had travelled to Nepal, West Hindustan and lower Burma. Many of his specimens are now housed in Kew Gardens alongside Banks's.

We now know this species was collected from Bhutan and we classify it under the species Valeriana wallichi.

Just to recap then. Jones had the roots correct as Nardostachys, but the leaf and flowers belonged to Valeriana wallichii which we now also know as Patrina.

Genus

Now, the common thread amongst these people was they struggled to put the plant into any particular genus. It transpired eventually this was because it did not exist.

Augustin Pyramus de Candolle was a Swiss botanist who eventually began a line of four generations of a family who dedicated their very existence to classification of plants. In 1830 De Candolle erected the Nardostachys genus for True Jatamansi and used the binomial "Nardostachys jatamansi" based on Patrina jatamansi (also known as Valeriana jatamansi sensu D.Don non Jones).

He added a second species *grandiflora* based on other Wallich material made available to him that had been originally found in Kumaon.

In 1975 German Botanist Dr Flocke Weberling revisited the genus notes and considered that all species along the Indo and Sino Himalayas should be included. Namely:

Nardostachys grandiflora DC (Which is the plant we use in aromatherapy)

Nardostachys Chinensis batalin (Used in Chinese medicine)

Nardostachys gracilis kitamura

All fall under the umbrella classification *Nardostachys jatamansi.*

So...

Our spikenard oil is taken from Nardostachys Jatamansi which also falls under the pseudonym *Nadostachys grandiflora.* However, *wallichi* (also sometimes referred to as Patrina), (under de Copella's guidance) falls under the same classification.

Recent thought had been that these were all the same plant, having different chemotyping due to their soil conditions. Recent research disputes that and places them as separate species. I can't help but wonder if, when Dioscorides says the plant that grows in the interior of the mountain is superior, he is speaking of wallichii and in fact this is the Nard of the Ancients, but of this I can provide no proof.

Botany

Nardostachys grandiflora DC or *Nardostachys jatamansi DC* belongs to the family Valerianaceae. Botanical classification of the plants is given below.

- Kingdom : Planate
- Division : Mangnoliophyta

- Class : Mangnoliopsida

- Order : Dipsacales

- Family : Valerianaceae

- Genus : Nardostachys

- Species : Jatamansi

- Botanical name : Nardostachys jatamansi DC

- Part used : Rhizomes, Rhizomes oil

Synonyms

N. jatamansi DC., N. chinensis, Fedia grandiflora WALL., Nardostachys gracilis KITAM., Patrinia jatamansi D. DON, Valeriana jatamansi auct. non JONES, Valeriana jatamansi sensu D. DON (BHATTARAI in litt. 2005, GOVERNMENT OF INDIA 1997, JAIN 1994, LANGE & SCHIPPMANN 1999, SCHIPPMANN in litt. 1997).

Local names

English : Nard, spikenard

Bhutan : Spang spos

India akashamansi, amritajata, balacharea, balachhada, balachhur, balchir, baluchar, bhutajata, bhutakeshi, bhutijatt, chakravartani, gandhamansi, gauri, hinsra, jadamansi, janani, jatala, jatalasi, jatamashi, jatamansi, jatamashi, jatavali, jati, jatilam jetamansi, kaichhad, kanuchara, keshi, khasambhava, kiritini, kravyadi, krishnsjata, kukulipot, laghumanshi, limasha, mansi, mansini, mashi, masi, massi, mata, mishika, misi, mrigabhaksha, nahni, nalada, niralemba, parvatavasini, peshi, peshini, pichachi, pishata, putena, sevali, shvetakeshi, sukshamajatamansi, sukshmapatri, sumbul, tamasi, tapasvini, behini

Nepal: bhulte, jatamansi, naorochi, naswan, pangbu, panghphoie,

Confusion in identification: Cites Appendix reads: There is disagreement regarding the similarity in appearance of the rhizomes of N. grandiflora and those of Valeriana jatamansi. The supporting statement of the 1997 proposal to include Nardostachys grandiflora in CITES Appendix II considered that the rhizomes of Valeriana jatamansi and V. officinalis look "superficially more or less alike" and that careful examination was required in order to distinguish them from each other (GOVERNMENT OF INDIA 1997). This point was supported by RAO (in litt. 1997). However, BHATTARAI (in

litt. 2005) argues that the species are not similar in *appearance,*
noting that while the rhizomes of N. grandiflora are covered with
hairs, the rhizomes of Valeriana jatamansi are completely hairless.
As a result, although the two species are used for similar purposes,
e.g. incense, he does not believe they are used as adulterants for each
other. AMATYA (in litt. 2005) similarly considers it unlikely that
the species are confused, like BHATTARAI, noting the difference in
their morphology and distribution (V. jatamansi is a temperate
rather than an alpine species).

Social Context

We spoke of the founding fathers of Unani in Rose Goddess Medicine. But I think here it requires us to look deeper at the societal context and religious beliefs that first inspired that medicine. In this book that medicine has an important place, not least because its roots lie in Graeco-Roman medicine and took its influences from Ayurveda, but also because the background helps us to understand the factions going on between the tribes and how the strife may eventually have lead to spreading of what potentially is the most important of the Hebrew and Hindu drugs.

It has its roots in Arabia, and when we meet the Phoenix later, you will discover that he too was from the same country. But, I asked myself, did I know where Arabia, the romantic land of Scheherazade and Aladdin was. I realised I did not.

Arabia was the region between the Yemen and the borders of Syria and Iran. The oldest evidence of people occupying this area dates back to around 3500BC when the Semites moved into Arabia and from there, we refer to this nation as the Sumerians. Those who settled in the south were referred to as the Babylonians and those who headed north, we know as the Assyrians. The Assyrian Empire was followed by a succession of Persian empires: the Achaemenids, Parthians and

Sassanids. There were three types of communities of these people, they were nomadic (Bedouins), agricultural and also there were urban settlers too.

The Arab world was greatly influenced by the Byzantine and Sassanian empires that surrounded their lands. These were extremely highly developed by this period. The art, the knowledge, the architecture of the late Roman periods could not help but permeate into other cultures. Alongside these ideas, Christian and Jewish religions began to trickle into the settlements too.

The medicine they practiced in these lands was understood as a relief of pain, either by themselves or by some external factor and by utilising some manner of their natural resources - so that might be air, heat, light or water, and probably some type of herb, spice or animal matter. This was the beginning of empirical medicine as we know it today.

Their medicine was practiced by three types of healer. These were the physician, the priest and the sorcerer or magician. Evidence of medicine dates back to the very earliest times, and was usually based on some degree of superstition or magic. Often there was the idea of a deity making some kind of intervention.

Incense

Over time then, it because necessary to establish a way of communing with their respective gods. Mysticism and faith began to take form and the idea that plants may be able to facilitate this conversation began to take hold.

An idea forms in the collective unconscious that scent lies somewhere between spirit and matter and can also influence cause and effect. In other words that fragrance can open a portal to instigate some kind of change.

Never more than in the case of incense was this true. Somehow the fragrance of the smoke was seen to mediate and to infuse the inner world with the outer world. The fumes were the required manner to connect the heavenly world with the earthly one. Most importantly that the fragrances were of the gods; that they emanated from them, but also that these perfumes had the ability to return *to* their source taking prayers and messages with them.

So the rites in the temple became ever more complex and sensory:

- The sound of the chant in juxtaposition to the silence of meditation.
- Statues ritually anointed and adorned with perfumes.

- Oils and unguents being used in ceremony. The fragrance of religion was both of communion but also commemoration of ancestral victories won and heartache from the nation's past.

Religion and medicine become inextricably linked.

One of the most famous incenses in history was burned in the City of the Sun, Heliopolis (also known as Hyperion.) The most famous Egyptian fragrance, kyphi, meaning "welcome to the gods", induced hypnotic states. Resins were burned in the morning, myrrh at noon and kyphi at sunset in an offering to the sun god, Ra.

Recipe for Kyphi By Rufus of Ephesus

(1st Century AD) Via Damocrates, Via Galen

Base: 90 g Raisins with skin and pips removed

               A little wine

               Sufficient honey

Gum Resins 90g Burnt resin

               45g nails of bdellium

Herbs   45g Camel Grass

33g sweet flag

11g Pure Cyperus grass

4 g saffron

11g spikenard

2 semis aspalathos

Spices: 15g Cardamom

11g   good cassia

Galen tells us the kyphi was be taken (that is internally rather than inhaled) as an antidote to snakebite. In Egypt, magic, religion, medicine, pharmacology, cosmetics, and chemistry was combined into one science. This was to become the norm through many different cultures

In 476AD, the Roman Empire fell. The civilisation, which had depicted its apotheosis with the symbol of a Phoenix, came to an end after almost a thousand years of rule. Where Europe went into cultural decline, the Arab world continued to focus its energies into understanding plant medicine and alchemy more deeply.

So, gather up you spice kit and follow the Phoenix across the sand dunes to his ancestral home. Watch, as he perches discretely out of view and begins his angelic song. Notice,how beneath him an apothecary is working a mortar and pestle and creating some mystical medicine for you to discover. Let's see who this ancient healer might have been and what we know about how he used our enigmatic jatamansi. Is he creating a perfume, a medicine and ointment or incense? And when we discover that will it lead us to being any closer to understanding what it was for?

Perfume

Horace gives us one of the greatest insights in the Nard of the Ancients, because his passages demonstrate just how favoured Nard was as a *perfume* as well as a medicine. From his works we get a real sense of a real high end bit of luxury kit. *Unguentum nardinum* was absolutely the gift *de rigueur* at parties, baths and feasts. When he is speaking to his brother poet, Virgil, we hear that in return for a very large vessel of wine, a small onyx box of Nard can be traded.

In *Odes* 4.12 he invites Virgil to his party on the condition that he brings a bottle of Nard with him:

"If you would drink a cup of choice wine at my house, bring a flask of precious nard with you. It will draw forth the wine bottle that lies in the Sulpician Vaults"

The vaults were heavily guarded communal wine caves at the foot of Aventine Hill. It was used by the wealthiest landowners to store their wine collections. Horace assures Virgil he will go and pick out a choice bottle of expensive wine as long as he can be relied upon to bring the precious Nard as a method of payment. It was a most appropriate gift for a guest to bring as thanks for an evening of hospitality.

Perfume had a very different context in the world of antiquity. Yes, people still wore it for adornment as they do today, but it had far wider uses. Remember, where we think of a spritz of Guerlain, perfumes such as Foliatum, Malabathron and Nard were oils to be anointed onto the body.

Perfumes played an enormous part in the Roman pastime of bathing. After taking the water, they were anointed, both publicly and privately. This anointing also took place after taking exercise at the gymnasium. It was the function of the patron to ensure there was always ample unguentum for the athletes.

They perfumed everything, from clothes and skin to their horses and dogs. Poets such as Horace found it shocking and obscene yet patricians saw it as a symbol of wealth and status and would clearly gauge a man's standing by the fragrances used in his home.

They were used at festivals and feast. Perfumes were sprayed around during processions (Remember Cleopatra and her perfumes emanating from the barge as she went to meet Mark Anthony?) Egyptians, Romans and Greeks alike all believed that the gods wished to be perfumed and would anoint idols, statues and altars in order to curry favour from a certain deity. We often refer to Theophastrus' work *Of Odors* as source material, but it was simply one of *many* wonderful works written by him. In "Characters" he depicts a pious and reverent man as anointing sacred stones that had been placed at the crossroads.

In the book, *Tastes of the Byzantine,* A. Dalby details an edict written by Leo VI, later to become known as The Wise, in 900AD that regulated practices in the Istanbul spice markets.

"Every perfumier shall have his own shop and not invade another's. Members of the guild are to keep watch on one another to prevent the sale of adulterated products. They are not to stock poor quality goods in their shops: a sweet smell and a bad smell do not go together.

They are to sell pepper, spikenard, cinnamon, aloeswood, ambergris, musk, frankincense, myrrh, balsam, indigo, dyers herbs, lapis lazuli, fustic, storax, and in short any article used for perfumery or dying.

The stalls shall be placed in a row between the milestone and the revered icon of Christ that stands above the Bronze arcade, so that the aroma my waft upwards and at the same time fill the vestibule of the Royal Palace"

Perfumes were vital at funerals, which we will look at more in depth in a moment and also in medicines which were so closely aligned that it sometimes seemed that fragrance and medicine were to all intents and purpose the same thing.

There is a passage in Galen's *In Antidotes,* where he criticizes perfume makers saying their knowledge of plants was insufficient and the antidotes they prepared were inefficacious.

This was because perfumers often encroached on physicians work, and likewise physicians liked to dabble with scents. The Hippocratic Corpus is a collection of 60 medical writings dating from the 1st Century AD; the work is strongly associated with Hippocrates, although it is not certain whether or not it was written by him.

In this work every perfume is written in the gynaecological section of the book. Clearly the writer gave the perfumes medical prowess, but also related this mode of healing only to womankind. Certainly Hippocratic physicians would dowse pessaries and make fumigations for treatment of the womb. Perfume making in the ancient world was almost paradoxical. The perfume merchants were seen as the highest order, holding rank equal to that of a doctor, by contrast being a perfume *maker*, a *seplasarius*, was a vocation of extremely low standing. In *"The Life of Heliogabulus"* (Emperor of Rome 218 – 222AD) we see the trade listed in the same status of *popinarius* (tavern keeper), *tabernarius* (shop keeper) and *leno* (brothel keeper). The costs of setting up a business needing presses and furnaces, not to mention the high value ingredients, however, would have been prohibitively high. This meant that, often, a wealthy family would start a business and put a slave in responsibility of it. But, given the massive profit returns a perfumery business could turn, many of these slaves found ways to improve their status a great deal. Given this then, one can see how the educated such as Galen may find these people encroaching on his patient list somewhat irksome.

One of the famous spikenard perfumes was *Megaleion*. Ancient Greek, and designed by Megallus, it is thought to be the world's first designer perfume. The wine and myrrh mixture was a complex set of ingredients including **Balanos oil** *Balanites aegyptiaca*, which was the base note of many Egyptian fragrances.

According to Dioscorides the recipe was Balanos oil, resin*, cinnamon, myrrh, carpobalsam, sweet flag, camel grass, wood balasam, costus, spikenard, amomum, although Pliny and Theophastrus describe slightly different recipes.

The Romans used spikenard in *Foliatum*, and *Natron* both of which were used to encourage hair growth and also in a scent named *Regelium*. Pliny describes Foliatum as the scent of rich women, and he discloses that it is largely manufactured in Palestine. He also explains the difference between the Nard fragrances of Foliatum as being made from the leaves and Spicatum from the spikes of the flower. Foliatum and Spicatum, Galen says, are both perfumes to be used to treat respiratory problems.

Pliny lists a recipe

Unguentus Nardinum Siva Foliatum

Indian nard, juncus (the leaves of Andropogon Seltwnmaims, L.), costus (the root of Aplotaxis aurieulata, DC.), amomum (the fruits of Amornum Cardamonzum, L.), myrrh (the gum-resin of Balsamodendron 111yrrlia, Nees), balm (the oleo-resin of Balsanzodendron Opobalsamum), ompliacium or olcum omphacinum (the oil expressed from unripe olives), and balaninurn (derived from Balanites wyyptiaca?). Dioscorides also remarks that malabathrum was sometimes added.

A flask of Foliatum was to be worn around the neck between the breasts. It was made of glass, gold or alabaster. In Israel and Palestine we see this same Foliatum referred to as Palyeton, and that because it was so popular, it became acceptable that this pendant of perfume could even be worn on the Sabbath.

Papers of rabbinic law give us an insight into just how loved nard was by Jews at the time of Christ. Drawing together notes from the Tosefta, which date to around the 2nd Century CE we can piece together a picture

Shabatt 62b tells us perfumes were added to flasks of spikenard. The spikenard was stored in a glass bottles (**Toseft Shabbat 8:20**) whose necks sometimes broke off (**Kelim 30: 4**) and when the bottle was opened the aroma escaped (**Abodah zara 35b**).

It seems likely that this amphora, worn between the breasts was the ointment used by Mary of Bethany to anoint Jesus.

My favourite rabbinic passage is from **Sanhedrin 108a** which tells us *"the fragrant spikenard oil could be appreciated even in the rubbish dumps."*

Thanks to the teachings of Rabbi Judah ben Baba we gain our first insight into why nard might have fallen out of favour. The martyred rabbi from the Second Century tells us "The perfumed spikenard oil was not used after the destruction of the Temple as a sign of national mourning". (Tosefta Sotah 15.9) (Tosefta Demai 1:26)

The fall of the Temple of Jerusalem, besieged and burned to the ground by the Romans, was in AD70.

There is one firsthand account of the siege, and this excerpt is from Josephus:

Most of the slain were peaceful citizens, weak and unarmed, and they were butchered where they were caught. The heap of corpses mounted higher and higher about the altar; a stream of blood flowed down the Temple's steps, and the bodies of those slain at the top slipped to the bottom.

No wonder no-one wanted to wear spikenard and risk being reminded....

Even if the rise of the Christianity did not put an end to the not only to the Nard's existence, but the perfumery trade as a whole, it could be said that it mortally wounded it. The Church believed that anointing oils and incenses should be preserved for the One True God. Even they could see the hygienic need for public bathing, but warned against promiscuity and of treatments involving oiling and massages administered by slaves. By the Middle Ages, the only people interested in taking up these expensive fragrances were the aristocracy and the church. The age of perfumery was, to all intents, over.

Or in hibernation, at least...

Anointing

This was a very common practice in early times. Anointing had four main functions.

One would anoint a visitor on their arrival as a symbol of honour and reverence but also in the desire to bestow some kind of good luck. One can see how it would be important to have something special to greet visitors of a higher status for example.

As mentioned before, anointing would take place on statue and sacred places too. Theocritus describes the consecration of the Planta tree at Sparta, in dedication to Helen of Troy for her wedding by the choir of the Lacedaemonian maidens. Celebrating her upcoming nuptials, but also lamenting their loss of a playmate, they hung consecrated wreaths of lotus flowers upon the tree, anointed it with costly spikenard and attached to it the dedication "Honour me, all ye"

Priests were anointed as a consecration to God and this probably stems from the story of the anointment of Aaron which we read in Exodus. It is thought the Oleo Santo, the Holy Chrism of the Greek Orthodox Church is still made from spikenard, and indeed the author of the protocol of the coronation of the Byzantine Emperor, Manuel II in 1391 tells us he had been anointed with a Myron of Spikenard.

Strabo the Roman geographer wrote of Alexander: *"His army used spikenard and myrrh for tent covering and bedding, thus at the same time enjoying sweet odor and a more healthy air"* . (Schoff makes an interesting point here. You will remember how Arrian had also described the grass being trampled by Alexander's retinue. Another problem arises with   =the standard translation, because there is no way that nardostachys could grow in the desert soil. It likes moisture too much. It seems likely that our Andropogon friend may have crept up on us here again.)

Nard became quite an obsession to Alexander, it seems, after he had stolen the ointments and cosmetics from the Persian King Darius III after his defeat at the battle of Issus in November 333BC.

The monarch anointed himself with *"an ointment composed of the fat of lions, palm wine, saffron, and the herb helianthes, which was considered to increase the beauty of the complexion."* Darius loved this ointment and took it everywhere with him even into battle, thus giving Alexander the opportunity to cease it and perhaps, one wonders giving him edge because Darius suspected it might give him some kind of competitive advantage. In Alexander's haul was also the **Royal Ointment** of the Parthian kings who ruled from 247BC – 248AD. Parthia later became Persia and now is modern day Iran. Previously it had been the lands of Assyria.

Pliny, in the first century related the ingredients of **Regale Unguentum as:** *henna, ben (myrobalan), putchuk, amomum, cinnamon, comacum (unidentified), cardamom, spikenard, zatar, myrrh, cassia, gum storax, ladanum, balsam, calamus, ginger-grass, tejpat, serichatum (unidentified), thorny trefoil, galbanum, saffron, nut grass, marjoram, cloves, honey and wine.*

It is difficult for historians to date the actual usage of this ointment exactly, since Pliny gives no indication of when it was used. Statuettes of the Parthians of the period do show them as having the red staining that henna would cause, so it seems likely that the paint was used as body art in much the same was as we still use it today. They must have looked and smelled hugely imposing and impressive. In the British Museum is housed, an Assyrian bas-relief that depicts a royal procession from Nimrud in 865 BCE. Traces of red colorant still remain on the soles and toes of the king and of some of his courtiers.

This stash of aromatic lovelies had a profound effect on Alexander and he began to collect fragrant ingredients from everywhere. Censers would dispense fragrant smoke in his tent at all times. He commenced collecting specimens of plants from all over the Empire and then to send them back to Athens. The collection was later to become the Athens Botanical Gardens. As Alexander became fixated with his ingredients, Roman and Greek interest into aromatic plants also began to swell.

Funeral Rites

Bodies were also anointed ready for burial.

Bringing flowers to the grave was a solemn affair held in the deepest esteem by the Romans. You may recall we discussed the Rosalia in *Rose Goddess Medicine*, where roses would be placed on the grave on the Day of The Dead, or perhaps also violets. In fact Ovid tells us, he *only* sees violets, but one poet, Ausonius, casts a different view point, stressing the importance of other fragrances and flowers, such as the rose, spikenard, and balsam. His epitaph reads, "*Sprinkle my ashes with pure wine and fragrant oil of spikenard: Bring balsam, too, stranger, with crimson roses. Tearless my urn enjoys unending spring. I have not died, but changed my state*".

At first glance one might suspect that this is his *own* epitaph, but no, Ausonius made a very nice living writing epitaphs for fallen heroes. More, Roman graves were constructed with pipes in which libations could be delivered into the grave. Often a tube would be placed into a broken or buried amphora so that the liquid, be it of wine or nard, could mingle with the remains of the dead, whether cremated or inhumed. The oils (macerations rather than essential oils, naturally) were as much to hide the smell of decomposition and to repel insects as to give thanks and blessing for their lives.

Medicine

The worlds of perfume, incense and medicine all so closely intertwine, it is impossible to separate them. I am reminded of how in the Yemen, when a baby is born, the women gather in a room, burn frankincense and the baby is wafted over the fumes to purify and strengthen it. Medicine? Possibly.

How did some of the authorities of the period use Indian Spikenard?

Abulcasis

Al Zahrawi (936AD) is thought of as the greatest surgeon of the Arab race. You may see his name Latinicised to *Abulcasis* or sometimes to *Alsaharavius.* He speaks of the benefits of *"Al-adhan"* which means the **fatness or oiliness that can be extracted from certain substances by pharmaceutical process.** Examples he uses are olives, sesame, eggs and wheat. These were used in treatments of diseases, externally by rubbing them on, or internally by drinking them.

He describes how certain ingredients can be added to the *Al adhan* to improve its therapeutic healing. These are roses, jasmine, lilies of the valley, cloves, cardamom, dill, thyme and our spikenard. What we see him preparing is a very ancient aromatherapy massage oil!

Troches were an important part of Unani medicine. They are sweetie tablets to be sucked. At the end of this chapter is a link to a document of extra recipes I found from Victorian England for you to download if you wish. You will see these recipes we see from Graeco- Roman times endured and were still very much in use in England in the nineteenth century.

Recipe for Rose Troches

Of blood in the stomach and the ailments thereof caused from the pouring in of yellow bile. Take of the red rose flowers, the root of glycyrrhizza, whose top parts removed, red sandalwood, yellow sandalwood, barberry bark, melilot, the pulp of melon seeds, mastic, spikenard, yellow amber, white traganth, white chalk, Persian mannam & safran.

Grind the drugs, sift and knead them together in dandelion water. Make them into tablets, the weight of each tablet dr i.

The dosage is one tablet to be taken with 4 oz of dandelion or black morel.

For morning sickness, Abulcasis directs using plasters containing the oil of spikenard, mastich, quinces, wormwood and the like or a vessel filled with hot water to be applied over the stomach. Pomegranate seeds should be held in the mouth and the patient should take gentle exercise and abstain from all sweet things.

Interestingly, Galen and Aetius account for morning sickness in the same way. They say that as the menstrual fluid is suppressed, a determination of it takes place to the stomach, until the foetus becomes large enough as to consume it.

Avicenna

Avicenna gives spikenard the name *Simbalath* in his Materia medica. The exact translation is Spica nigra and he distinguishes between several kinds. The first he calls *alnardin* or *nardin*.

Most people assert that he probably means Indian spikenard, but in reality it is more likely he means *celtic* nard, (valerian because he calls it *Nardus Romani orbit* referring to its European roots.

Subsequently he does refer to the **spikenard of Asiatic origin,** of which **there are several kinds.** These are Indian spikenard growing in different places and as such their origin affects how good they are (because of soil composition, presumably, but also perhaps because there are different chemotypes).

One of the properties he suggests, is **using spikenard to aid the eyelashes to grow,** and as an **antidote to the eyelashes falling out.**

My Latin has come on leaps and bounds with this book. A new word I have learned is collyria. These are specifically Roman seals used to label eye washes and eye medicines.

A number of these have been found spread around the Empire, not least one found in 1849 in Kenchester which is the village where I spend most of my Sunday afternoons buying new tropical fish! It is just outside Leominster about twenty minutes from my home in Ludlow and is the ancient Roman site of Magnis. These collyria are rare in Britain and this one from Kenchester is one of only two found here.

It is engraved on four sides. Unfortunately only three sides are legible now. These are

- Anicetum (Aniseed, perhaps)
- Nard (You know the drill)
- Chloron (Eye Wash)

The maker, the oculist, was one Titus Vindaci Ariovisti, the only named Roman we know of in Herefordshire.

In a 1926 paper in the British Journal of Opthalmologists the translation of Anicetum is challenged (wouldn'yt ya know!) Anicetum can also be translated as "unconquered". Oriabasius described an Anicetum Collyrium as comprising as red copper, menlock, henbane, spikenard and frankincense and as being good for carbuncles!!!

Antidotes

This idea of an antidote we saw with Galen and his eyelashes was very powerful. It is as if, providing one could identify just the right plant to appease the gods, then one could switch off the pain. Even Galen's most famous treatise was called "On Antidotes".

Hippocrates rarely has more than 6 ingredients in his antidote recipes but Scribonius Largus often has far more than 7, some as many as 20 bits and pieces.

Marcianus

We hear that the most potent antidote was that of the physician, Marcianus, whose medicinal masterpiece has a gut blowing 40 ingredients many of which are exotic and rare.

*"Antidote of the physician Marcianus, which is called **telea** (meaning "is perfect" in Greek) because it lacks of nothing. This single [antidote] works against all [ills] against which all the best antidotes work. This antidote used to be compounded for Augustus Caesar.*

8 denarii of cinnamon, 6 denarii of amomum, 25 denarii of black cassia, 16 denarii of saffron, 5 denarii of rush, 5 denarii of frankincense, 2 denarii of white pepper, 10 denarii of myrrh, 10 denarii of long pepper, 10 and a half denarii of Indian spikenard, 16 denarii of celtic nard, 6 denarii of dried rose , 2 denarii of white costus, 4 denarii opobalsumum, half a denarius of Cyrenaic silphium, or one denarius of Syrian, 6 denarii of cassidony, 5 denari of gentian, 4 denari of root of sharp clover, or 3 denari of the seed of this plant, 12 denarii of scordium, 5 denarii of germander, 2 denarii of hazelwort, 2 denarii of sweet flag, 32 denarii of valerian, 2 denarii of copper ore, 12 denarii of dittany, 3 denarii of drops of ammoniacum, two times the semis if agaricum [a fungus], 20 drops of balsam, 6 denarii and a half of parsley, three times a semis of wild rue, three times a semis of fennel seeds, 4 denarii of Cretan daucus, 2 denarii of anise, 2 denarii of Ethiopian cumin, 5 and half denarii of turnip seeds, 3 denarii of wild mustard seeds, 2 denarii of fresh blood of female duck, dried blood of male duck, 3 denarii of dried blood of male kid, 6 denarii and a half of dried blood or turtle, 3 denarii of dried blood of male goose, and a sufficient amount of Attic hone. It works against everything."

I should think it does. What was it Michael Caine said?

"You're only supposed to blow the bloody doors off....!"

Heavens a-plenty, he wasn't messing about was he?

Also did you notice what I did? Celtic Nard (16 denarii) and valerian (32 denarii) are in the same recipe and so they couldn't have been the same thing. I wonder if I am the first person to spot that?!

Anyway. Dried goat blood anyone? No?

Let's move on then.

Hippocrates mentions spikenard twice in his *Hippocratic Corpus*, both times for gynaecological complaints.

Galen

Earlier we spoke of the distinction between the nard perfumes *spicatum*, made of the spikes and *foliatum* of the leaves. **In both cases Galen recommends inhaling them for respiratory diseases.**

He makes a distinction between _cosmetics_ which he refers to as _heating agents_, and thus being medicinal in nature and *commotics* which he sees as the **simple art of adornment**.

"For more vigorous heating agents, add euphorbia to oil and all pepper based preparations. Anoint the forehead and nostrils with perfumes, particularly iris, marjoram and spikenard oil. Cosmetic products are heating agents, especially those exorbitant perfumes that rich women use, known as foliata and spicata.

Galen speaks in his book *Of Antidotes* of the Poison of Mithradian.

Mythradian

Greek King Mithridates VI of Pontus (135–63 BC) was a charismatic ruler. He inspired fear and respect across the Near East. So terrified was Mithradates, of being poisoned that he took daily doses of his own concocted poison in an effort to build up a resistance to any future attempts. Now it has to be said that Galen often utilises the phrase "they say" seemingly in an effort to distance himself from the story perhaps because he doesn't exactly trust it. That would seem wise since historical accounts show Mithradates eventually committed suicide...by drinking poison. Doesn't seem to add up really does it?! Either that or it was like his version if ripping up early drafts that he thought were rubbish, only to find actually, he made fairly good poisons...dunno.

Nevertheless, Galen relates part of the recipe as *bdelion, galbanum, cardamom, cassia, cinnamon, costus-root, nard, opobalsamum, pepper and storax;* Like me, another ambassador of the whack it all in and see what happens, approach, I think!

Good lad.

Galen's use of Nard on Marcus Aurelius

Just before we move on, I thought I would tell you how Galen came to be so revered as a surgeon. You remember how our

Marcus Aurelius was happily smacking taxes on everything containing Nard? Well he smacked spikenard onto something else too.

In 176 Marcus Aurelius (MA) returned to Rome and was taken ill. He was surrounded by the doctors who travelled with him, who seem to be all fawning after him anxious that a fever may suddenly befall him. MA is in pain though, and none of their remedies seem to be making a blind bit of difference.

Galen had previously helped to heal Commodus and so he too was called to the bedside. It transpired that MA had taken oil of aloes and then followed it with his daily dose of, the then universal, antidote called *theriac*. Consequently when night came he was racked with colic and diarrhoea. The physicians around him watched the symptoms, took his pulse and looked in a puzzled manner at each other. Then they ordered rest and fed him porridge the next day. He would heal and then of course the next day he'd imbibe the offending antidote and the cycle would continue again.

The next day Galen was invited to stay overnight at the palace to oversee the strange symptoms. He discretely listened and watched the physicians discussing their strange machinations but said nothing. They pressed him to take his pulse and at first he stalls saying he does not know the patient well enough to understand what a normal pulse might look like, but when pressed simply guesses at one. He then announces that there is no problem with fever, but that the Emperor is suffering from indigestion "His stomach" he says" was oppressed by the food he has eaten" (Probably as a veiled criticism of this never ending cycle of porridge!).

Think for a second how brave a step this was.

The court physicians are utterly convinced there is something dire afoot. They are afraid enough to call someone from outside their inner sanctum....and when he comes he tells the Emperor- someone he has never treated before and thus with whom he holds no reputation- that this killer disease is something as trivial as indigestion. He then prescribed wool soaked in warm nard. He also tells the Emperor that for an ordinary person he would have suggested a therapy of wine and pepper because of the prohibitive cost of the nard. Impressed Aurelius uses both the wine and pepper blend along with the nard and quickly feels much better – *a pad of scarlet wool, soaked in nard, applied to the rectum.*

Aurelius then famously says "We have one physician only" presumably having an irritated snipe at the three pokers and prodders "and he is completely noble". From then on Galen is always referred to as "The First among Physicians.

The Dynameron

You may recall us speaking about The Dynameron, in Rose Goddess Medicine. The document by Nikolaos Myrepsos, a 13th Century physician at the Byzantine court of John III Doukas Vatatzes at Nicaea dates to the 13th Century. It is a beautifully illuminated manuscript detailing hundreds upon hundreds of antidotes.

The translation by the Greek scholars in 2013 was no mean feat and I am interested to see that they list the most important Nard of the ancients as *Nardostachys jatamansi (D. Don)*.

It appears in 106 recipes under several names: *nardostachys* (in 92 recipes), *nardos* (in 10 recipes), *nardos of India* (in 3 recipes), *nardou stachys* (in one recipe).

The works shows how Myrepsos used nard as a perfume, incense but mainly as a sedative. The root was a primary ingredient in medications created to treat diseases of:

- Liver
- Kidney
- Gynaecological bleeding
- Inflammations of the uterus and abdomen
- Flatulence

- Heart disease
- Urination
- Constipation
- Diarrhoea
- Jaundice.

Brace yourselves...For comparison, for the scholars of us who are now in the know...

The name *nardos celtice* is found in 21 recipes and in two recipes.

The name *nardos of Syriais* cited in 12 recipes and the name *stachos* in 97 recipes. Both are identified as *Patrinia scabiosifolia or Golden Valerian.*

Three more related names are found in the text, *nardou rhiza* (i.e. root of nard) *nardos agria* (which means wild nardos) both cited once and *fou* cited in 16 recipes. *Nardou rhiza* is identified to *Valeriana officinalis L.,* while *nardos agria* and *fou* are thought to be either to *Valeriana dioscoridis Sm.* A very pretty pink flower known as Italian Valerian, or to a similar looking plant *Valeriana italic Lam.*

Paulus Aegenita

Paulus Aegenita was a seventh century Byzantine physician. In his work he mentions spikenard often. Here are some of my choicest favourites.

Preservatives of hoary hairs and other compositions for dying them black

(For making the hair curled, and for dying it from Cleopatra)

Of the oil of unripe olives, three sextarii, or spikenard dr.j. of unguis aromaticus (sweet hoof?) dr iv; of schoenanth dr iv

Boil with oil, and separately pound and dissolve carefully one ounce of the juice of acacia in wine.

He is very clear that spikenard should be used to take care of the teeth. He warns caution in of eating anything too hard, like dried figs that have been boiled in honey, and advises that teeth should always be cleaned after supper.

He tells us that Rhases suggests *Of hartshorn, the seeds of tamarisk, of cyperus and spikenard. Take the salt of a gem, let it be pulverised and the teeth rubbed with it.*

Also, he says Celcus recommends spikenard for the treatment of colic. He recommends principally dry fermentation, friction of the hands and feet and dry cupping. He also speaks of a medicine which he names as the "colic composition" made of poppy tears, pepper, anise, castor, spikenard and myrrh.

You'll be relieved to hear that he comes to our rescue on days we suffer **putrid smell and sweating of the armpits.**

He prescribes:

Of liquid alum, of amomum, of myrrh and of spikenard, or each dr.iv; titrate with wine and use.

Incidentally all the authorities of the period seem to concur with these recommendations for this complaint. Mix a combination of astringents and aromatics.

The Geniza Collection

The Geniza Collection comprises 193,000 fragments of medieval manuscripts, mainly Hebrew, Judeo-Arabic, Aramaic and Arabic. Found in the Ben Ezra Synagogue in Fustat, Old Cairo in 1896-97 by Solomon Schechter and his colleague Charles Taylor, the collection gives an unrivalled perspective into the societal, religious and pharmacological traditions of their time. Some of the fragments date back to as early as 9th and 10th Century. I am grateful to Efraihim Lev for his wonderful cataloguing and commentary.

Here we see spikenard used in several ways, most often as electuries. These are powders, mixed with honey, syrup or some other confection as a means to sweeten the pill. This is the medieval version of a "Spoonful of sugar makes the medicine go down..."

Each recipe begins in the same manner

In your name, O Merciful One....

Description of a musk remedy that is good for tremors, and palpitations and loneliness

Take mastic and cinnamon and cloves and spikenard, seven pills and nutmeg and cubeb and lesser cardamom and sedge and aloeswood, and citron leaves and seeds of sweet basil [that] strengthens buds of cloves and basil seeds and dry sweet marjoram and wild thyme and ginger and long pepper and cucumber the weight of ten dirhems.

Pearl and coral and amber and raw silk and red behen and Indian laurel and grind ten dirhems of each, along with pure musk, two daniqs and mix after grinding and sifting and knead with honey of candies cherubic myrobalan

Beneficial if God wills

Cherubic is *Terminalia chebula* which is even now being researched for its ability to purge the body of toxins amongst other properties.

For reference a dirhem was a unit of weight used across North Africa, the Middle East, and Persia, with varying values.

Hibaï Allâh ibn Ṣāʻid Ibn al-Tilmīd

Hibaï Allâh ibn Ṣāʻid Ibn al-Tilmīd was a 12th century Christian physician in Baghdad. The doctor, who was also a skilled poet and musician worked his was way up to be chief physician of the hospital and the Physician to the Caliph, Al-Mustadi.

He wrote several works, the most important being *Al-Aqrābādhīn al-Kabir*. This important pharmacopeia was to become the standard way of treating patients throughout the Arabic civilisation. It replaced the works of Sabur Ibn Sahl which had been the standard method of treating people for 300 years prior. *Aqrabadin* is the seminal text to understand medieval medicine and also the medicine of the west which took its lead from this.

He has a lovely recipe using spikenard contained therein:

A hospital stomachic which is useful against incontinence by retaining it.

Cyperus, Indian spikenard, French lavender, frankincense and the bark of its tree, acorns and the inner skins of their cups and cumin in equal parts. A potion may be made using one mitqual of it in the morning and just as much on the evening.

A mitqual is the old Arabic measure used to weigh precious commodities such as gold or saffron. Its modern day equivalent is 4.25g

The Syriac Book of Medicines

Thought to date from the 12th century, the Syriac Book is an overview of the school of thought that flourished in the Graeco Roman and Sassanian Periods.

It lists Nards as being:

A remedy for colds and congestive conditions of the head and body generally

- Sedative of nervous diseases
- Treatment of paralysis
- A remedy for consumption (that is tuberculosis to you and I)
- Abdominal congestion or ulceration
- Dropsy (remember oedema?)
- Inflammation of the liver and spleen
- Use on external plasters for reduction of inflammation

It is interesting to note that here, it was not seen as a nerve stimulant which given its close association with love charms one might expect that it might have been.

Spikenard Red Herrings

There have been loads of red herrings and close off cul-de-sacs of research in this book. The general concensus on my facebook page was that readers wanted to experience the research in its entirety, so here are a couple of the first ones.

In Arabia, they spoke of a perfume called Nadd.

Al- Nuwari was a 14th Century celebrated lawyer and historian and is considered to be the chief authority of the Muslim world at this time. He wrote the "Encyclopaedia of Human Knowledge which is broken down into five divisions: Heaven and Earth, Man, Animals, Plants and History. Contained therein are a number of recipes of two standard ointments *Ghaliya* and Nadd. (Note Nadd, not Nard, which may or may not be important.)

He says:

"Tamimi mentions different sorts such as the Nadd Al-musta'ini which was prepared for the Abbisside Caliph Musta'in billah al-abbas

50 parts Indian Aloe, Same quantity of Tibetan musk, 150 parts blue shihir ambergris, 3 parts Riyaddhi camphor.

Aloe musk and camphor are ground with a mortar and pestle and the musk pressed through a silk cloth. Ambergris is dissolved in a jar or vase with the ground ingredients stirred in. It is then poured onto a marble plate and then cut into bars.

Did you spot the deliberate mistake? No spikenard anywhere in that recipe, and actually Schoff was able to show many where spikenard was not included, but ambergris always was. So the question of course must be...is *Nadd* of the Arabic world, the same as the *Nard* of Iranian and Indian worlds? So he looked up the etymology in a couple of dictionaries. The English/Arabic dictionary Havas simply says that *Nadd / Nidd* means Perfume. Not very helpful, but when he looked up in another one called Freytag, the listing said "Nadd – The perfume of ambergris, musk and aloeswood, referred to by others as Ambergris".

Not spikenard.

We must hope for the sakes of research and for our sanity, that Nadd was a different thing and should not be confused with Nard.

If you are not bored yet, feel free to enjoy red herring two. I have put together a little pamphlet of Victorian remedies I have found on the journey, but I am fairly certain that although they list spikenard, they cannot be referring to our same Nardostachys jatamansi. We know that Granville showed specimens of Nardostachys to many eminent pharmacists in London and **none of them recognised it**. We have to ask ourselves then, how can this be so? If it is listed in so many recipes, and important ones too, how is it they don't know what it is? The only conclusion I can draw is that they were using valerian, maybe lavendula latifolia (spike lavender) or may be stoechas (French lavender). It seems unlikely that these recipes were made up with Nardostachys.

One last suggestion might be a plant "Spignel". The reason I suggest it, is that I kept coming across information saying that spikenard had a ruling planet of Venus. This seemed to be strange to me, completely the opposite of what I would suspect. Then I found what I think might be the source, in Culpepper.

But on closer examination, although he does ask for Indian Spikenard in some of his recipes and recommendations he has also written a monograph dedicated t "Spikenard". But it is not our plant. He talks about a plant he names as Spikenard or **Spignel.** Other English names include Baldmoney, (also Spiknel and Spikenel), or its botanical name is *Meum athamanticum.* This is a plant of the Apiacae family and smells a bit like angelica. It is not a plant I have seen, I don't think. It grows mostly in Scotland. His classification of this plant is

Venus and has very different properties to our Nardostachys. If this is the plant that the Victorian apothecaries were using then these Victorian recipes are obsolete to our study.

Nevertheless they are amusing to read so knock yourself out....

You can find the recipes at: https://buildyourownreality.leadpages.co/spikenard/

Chapter 2 The Spikenard of The Bible

Spikenard's old testament name is: שָׁבּוּלֶת נֵרְד

To the Hebrews and the Jews of today, spikenard is known as Shibolet Nard (Nard Spike) and is used as part of the festival of Passover.

Exodus

For a moment I want you to imagine yourself as a Hebrew, in the blazing heat of the Egyptian sun, toiling day and night building the glory of the Pharaohs, constructing idols to gods who are not your own. The garlic they feed you to keep you strong protects your physical body, but your mind still reels. You live in fear each day that yours might be the next family to be made example of. Threats of children being put to work if you do not move enough bricks ring in your ears. You collect more and more straw to make them, terrified of the outcome if you do not do so.

For 400 very long years it has been so.

You dare not imagine that it could be ever any different, and yet, there has always been a tale....

A prophecy perhaps,

Of a leader who will rise up, free you from bondage and will deliver you to the Promised Land.

But Goshen, the land given to the Hebrews, by Joseph when Jacob brought his people to safety under his son's rule, has become a heinous place. Now, far from being a home, it is the centre of a brick building workforce of two million slaves and every day the dream seems to slip further away.

But then one day he does appear. This man they call Moses. A Hebrew, who has been raised as Egyptian prince, fits the prophecy and he has the charisma and skills that make it seem like escaping the clutches of Rameses the Great might be something you could actually pull off.

You watch as plagues, floods, famine, disease ravages your country. You observe how the "Great" Pharaoh does nothing to help his people. You look on in dismay and disgust. You pray grateful thanks for the love and mercy of your Lord for sparing your children as he has killed the firstborn of every Egyptian man. Eventually you are persuaded to leave your home and flee this dreadful subjugation.

At the stroke of midnight of the day of 15 Nissan 2448 from Creation, you, along with 600,000 adult males, with women and children, leave Egypt to head for Mount Sinai. Regardless of the hell you leave behind, the prospect of your journey towards Canaan, a Promised Land is overwhelming.

You are to travel across deserts, through the wilderness, unsure of where your next meal will come from and always terrified that Egyptians are on your tail. When, *if*, you finally get there...what greets you in Canaan then? Inhabited by warring tribes, this place of Milk and Honey is itself a raging hotbed of political unrest. You could be easily wandering to your death.

The nights will be cold. The wind will ravage and as an Israelite, I am sure you would have felt absolutely alone.

Sacred Incense of The Israelites

Then, God spoke to Moses and instructed him to build the Tabernacle, a majestic tent, so that the Israelites could worship and be renewed in their faith. And on the altar of the Tabernacle, must burn an incense of sweet smelling perfumes to bring the people closer to their God.

Now The Old Testament tells us about four ingredients.

- *stacte* (נָטָף *nataf*) – which is generally thought to be **myrrh**
- onycha (שְׁחֵלֶת *shekheleth*) – Possibly some kind of sea shell, but also other suggestions have been

cistus/labdanum/rock **rose** or other sources suggest
cloves.

- **galbanum** (ה‎ַ‎ל‎ָ‎ב‎ַ‎נ‎ָ‎ה *khelbanah*)
- **frankincense** (ל‎ַ‎בֹ‎ו‎ָ‎נ‎ָ‎ה ז‎ַ‎ר‎ָ, *levonah zach*)

But if we leave Christian writings for a moment and visit the
Talmud, it tells us the *Qetoret* contained *eleven* spices. There
were seventy measures each of (1) balsam, (2) onycha, (3)
galbanum, and (4) frankincense. There were sixteen measures
each of (5) myrrh, (6) cassia, (7) spikenard, and (8) saffron.
There were twelve measures of (9) costus, three measures of
(10) aromatic bark, and nine measures of (11) cinnamon.

I am going to ask you now to put the book down. Go to the
spice cupboard or your oils box and see how many of these
ingredients you have. Gather them together and just take the
tops off and breathe....

Let's just experience the aromatherapy those poor, frightened
people must have felt as they entered that space...calming,
supporting, comforting....

Those wonderfully exotic fragrances transport us back to the
tent, to that heat, to the incense giving respite to the scourge of
the flies outside. To the calmness of the space where it is so
much easier to believe that God protects you.

That you are chosen...

That you are not alone; *that there can be miracles when you believe.*

The Bible speaks of spikenard several times, but the Talmud, and rabbinic writings, bring the history of spikenard into clearer focus. The *Pseudepigraphia* is a collection of Jewish works that date from between 300BC – 300AD. One of these works, the *Revelation of Moses*, thought to date to around the 2nd century AD, describes Adam and Eves' story from their expulsion from the garden to the end of their lives, including the tale from Eve's point of view.

Ancient Jewish documents describe the Revelation as being given to Moses, by the Archangel Michael at the same time as he was given the Ten Commandments.

Michael shows Moses how, some eighteen years and two months after their expulsion, Adam and Eve eventually conceived Cain and Abel.

The Revelation of Moses tells us: *And after this, Adam and Eve were with one another; and when they lay down, Eve said to Adam her lord: My lord, I have seen in a dream this night the blood of my son Amilabes, who is called Abel, thrown into the mouth of Cain his brother, and he drank it without pity. And he entreated him to grant him a little of it, but he did not listen to him, but drank it all up; and it did not remain in his belly, but came forth out of his mouth. And Adam said to Eve: Let us arise, and go and see what has happened to them, lest perchance the enemy should be in any way warring against them.*

Overcome with grief, Adam lay with Eve and they conceived Set, and then subsequently thirty more children who occupied the Earth in three parts. Adam became old and infirm and deeply upset and as his children gathered around him before he died, both he and Eve told the tale of how the Devil had spoken to them, through the mouth of the serpent, and how as they had eaten of the forbidden fruit, God had cast him out.

The Lord had cursed the land so it might always be labourious for Man to survive, and the angels were terrified for Adam. After pleading with God for mercy, Adam turns his efforts to the angels, and we hear:

Our father Adam wept at the gates of paradise and the angels said unto him "What wilt we do to thee, Adam". He then answered, "Behold, ye cast me out; therefore I entreat you to give me some sweet spices from Paradise, that when I am driven out of it I may offer a sacrifice to God that he may hear me". Then at the request of the angels God gave Adam leave to gather from the garden saffron and spikenard, sweet cane and cinnamon and other seeds for his support. Having gathered them, he left the garden and dwelt in the land.

This revelation, of course, sets the stage for the beginnings of the sacred incense that will become vital to the Israelites faith.

Charoset

Somehow spikenard seems to have deep connections to Passover. It's most famous event was reputed to happened just a few days before Passover. Earlier, we have this dreadful toil in Egypt, collecting straw, making bricks and then constructing gargantuan statues and architecture. Then God sent his plagues but when the first born child of the Hebrews was spared, the nation celebrated with Passover. Strangely, two very important 14th century documents, the Rothschild *Mazhoor* (Florence 1490) and the *Second New York Haggarda* (1454) have identical lists for their recipes for Charoset, the sacred meal to celebrate Passover and the emancipation of the Jews.

The instructions stipulate that it is necessary to use spices reminiscent of straw. Shibolet Nard and cinnamon are listed as examples. The charoset has vegetables as the main ingredient and should be made thickly to resemble the mud with which they worked.

Song of Solomon

Almost as famous as the anointing of Christ, is spikenard's place in the enigmatic and sensuous Song of Songs. It is an expertly written piece of poetic prose which has hidden depths. Whist you wouldn't flinch from reading it alongside your parents, on closer inspection it has undeniably erotic undertones. It is thought to have been written by a bridegroom for his bride as a pre-cursor and reassurance of the beauty of their first night together. As to who the author is, there is controversy. (Wouldn't you know?!) It seems fairly certain that even though Solomon is referred to by name, he is probably not responsible for it. At the end of the 3rd Century BCE, Aramaic began to replace the old Hebrew language and so linguistically the times do not match. There is a possibility that it may even have been Ancient Egyptian in origin and might actually have been a love poem of Ishtar and her sacred marriage to the god Tammud – her Gardener King. In the Ancient Babylonian tablets of the Epic of Gilgamesh we also see a similar idea of Ishtar and her love for Usallanu, also the Gardener King.

The Epic of Gilgamesh is the oldest poem in existence and it details how the priestess of Ishtar seduces the wild man Ednika into a weeklong sexual union, she teaches him the ways of the civilised man. This sacred union between deity and human is termed *heiro gamos,* it is one of the oldest practices of tantric union.

We know of some of the rites of the heiro gamos. That the priestess would lead the priest up the steps of the Ziggarat of Ur and when they reached the eighth layer, the stage had been laid out as a bedroom and there, the priest would anoint the the head of the priestess with spikenard. This was her crowning as deity.

The heiro gamos, was a very public display with processions and watchers of the union, and was to guarantee the health of the following year's harvest. The union of the rain god and the sun goddess was beloved for many centuries. We know it was practiced in Sumeria, Babylonia and Mesopotamia and also in Canaan, most pertinently through their god Ba'al..

In Christianity of course, the most famous of the heiro gamos is Mary and the Holy Spirit, but it became impossible for the Church to marry the idea of sexual union and the worshipful idolatry of goddesses like Isis, Innana, Ishtar or even of Ba'al which might be why we hear of the strangely unusual idea that the Mother of God was a virgin. (Of course, again, she might have been that too!)

The Song of Songs (note the idea of its being superlative, a little like the Holy of Holies) seems not to have any kind of literary construction as such. So one wonders: is it a song, is it a poem, or is it a collection of works? An anthology perhaps? There *is*, however, a theme.

The woman in the poem seems to be the instigator of the seduction. Both are extremely willing and full of anticipation for one another. The reader is invited into the union by way of the Jerusalem chorus, and these women urge the union on and on. At the end of each passage the woman bids the Jerusalem Chorus not to stir up love, such as hers ,until it is ready. This repetition becomes a theme through the song...wait...not yet...not yet. Extremely tantric naturally, but note how the presence of Jerusalem Chorus seems to demonstrate the idea of a procession or other people being involved in the union.

"A garden locked is my sister, my bride, A rock garden locked, a spring sealed up. Your shoots are an orchard of pomegranates. With choice fruits, henna with nard plants, Nard and saffron, calamus and cinnamon, With all the trees of frankincense, Myrrh and aloes, along with all the finest spices."

There is very much an idea of chastity, isn't there? It is fragrant, but locked and unvisited. Is the sacred union a virgin one I wonder?

Wilfred Schoff describes how the term Nard first appears in *Indian* writings in the Arthrarva Veda where it is mixed with honey and made into an ointment. Arthrarva is the fourth veda and the term means literally "knowledge". It is made up of 730 sanskrit hymns, 6000 mantras and comprises 20 books. About one sixth of it is the beautiful Rig Vedas, the love songs we explored in the Holy Basil book. Sometimes you might see this referred to as the "Book of Magic Formulas" and it probably dates somewhere between 1200-1000 BC. Again here, we have this sense of Nard being used for seduction.

"Nala" or "Nard" is also found in the *Aitareya* and the *Sankjayana Araya* as a prescription against bad dreams. In both cases it is spoken of as "wreath" or a garland"...which of course means that this time it cannot be relating to an ointment. This is most assuredly a plant.

In the passage we see mention of the *Asparas*. These are celestial nymphs revered in Hinduism and here the story speaks of the five asparas who are driven out by some herb. Each aspara has the name of a plant, for example we see guggulu which translates to Bdellium. So, here in these sacred texts we can trace something very special about the plant to some kind of magical being.

So when we read another line from Arthrarva "As India is possessed of glory and heaven-and-earth as the waters are possessed of glory in the herbs, so among all the gods may we, among all be glorious" we can see that the herb bestows magical powers onto the human race through their association with the plants.

In this case, particularly Nard or Nala has a connection with love and vigour and the uses of the drug were particularly aligned with the Mother Goddess.

It seems likely when we see very early Mohamedeen practices of anointing sacred spaces like the Ka'ba at Mecca and the Sacred Rock under the Temple of Jerusalem, that these ceremonies have their roots in using nard to celebrate the Mother Goddess.

The *Kausika Veda* is a ritual book connected from within the Arthrarva Veda which gives beautiful insights into the beliefs and practices of the ordinary Hindu, not least their terrors about demons in the world. Contained therein is a charm designed to attempt to assure the safety of the herd. Here Nard should be given to calves to drink while a priest performs a special ceremony.

Over time Nard became associated with rituals of great weight, namely marriages and funerals. For marriages it would be reserved for royalty and high status families. if for no other reason than its prohibitive costs.

Phyllarchus wrote about the ancient Greek world from 220-275BC, and although his writings have not survived, he is quoted as an authority by many other writers of antiquity. He is attributed with an antidote of a gift of a love charm which is not named but is thought to most likely pertain to Nard. It had been sent by **Chandragupta** Maurya, the first Emperor to unify Greater India to Seluclid empire. The Greek had decided to abandon the traditional customs and to mimic Solomon when he decided to take wives from all of the peoples under his dominion.

In *Liber Dicersarum Hacreseon*, Philastrus also mentions a special balm for marriage which had been lovingly prepared by the Indians of the Punjab. Here he relates how, unless the young couple had the balm sprinkled over them, their union was not deemed complete or compatible with Aphrodite's grace. Again here we have very strong connotations with Mother Goddess sect. Certainly there are echoes of the same idea of Nard as a ceremonial offering to the Goddess of Love we see in Song of Songs.

So Nard is a charm for weddings and for funerals. Both have associations with extreme emotions but from a primitive point of view we might think of the waxing and the waning of the moon, or Ishtar's descent into Hades, or initiation into something new; embracing the dark night of the soul to understand the true capabilities of spirit; invoking the feminine divine. We see the goddess initiation. Thus, of course in each case it is only right that there *should* be an anointing.

Transition...initiation....

There is a beautiful book called Sexual Secrets by Penny Slinger and Nick Douglas where they speak extensively about the ancient Tantric Rite of the Five Essentials which has spikenard at the very heart of the ritual. It might be that this predates the Arthrarvedic writings even, perhaps dating back to India's aboriginal Pre-Vedic peoples (Pre-1500BCE).

The ritual was a means of spiritual accomplishment through the male-female exchange. In Tantra the woman has "the rights". Her energy is seen as flowing, yielding, submissive and very much linked to femininity. Here, Goddess initiates god. After preparing offerings of food to Lakshmi, the man applies jasmine to his lover's hands, patchouli to her neck and cheeks, spikenard to her hair and musk to her vagina. In turn she rubs him all over with sandalwood.

Beautifully sensuous, and most unmistakably related, again, to the Mother Goddess.

It is almost irresistible, then, to think back to the leper's house and to that infamous woman of disrepute and her hair. Clearly the event was deemed to be something special, worthy of comment, because the story is told in each of the four gospels (albeit with slightly different details in each). These ideas which seem newly uncovered to us were part and parcel of the environment of the day. As Jesus was doused in this infamous love token, one cannot help but wonder what people thought they might have walked in on.

Chapter 3 New Testament

Its new testament name is νάρδοςε

Spikenard at His Birth

The most famous of all the Biblical tales of Nard must surely be his anointing by Mary of Bethany. There is much confusion over this, as the Magdelene was later to become branded as whore as the Church chose to align the two women (Later in 1969, they issued an edict to say there had never been any evidence to brand her thus.) There are also two different accounts of women anointing Christ and they often become confused. Mary of Bethany anointed him six days before Passover as the Sanhedrin had issued a warrant for Jesus's arrest. This is found in John 12.1-11; Matt. 26.6-13; Mark 14.3-9. In John we hear she anointed His hair and feet, but in Matthew and Mark, only his head.

The account of the "Sinful Woman" happens in Luke and seems to be some months, if not years, prior to his death. The Sinful woman may have been Mary, but the Bible does not tell us that she is.

When one of the Pharisees invited Jesus to have dinner with him, he went to the Pharisee's house and reclined at the table. [37] A woman in that town who lived a sinful life learned that Jesus was eating at the Pharisee's house, so she came there with an alabaster jar of perfume. [38] As she stood behind him at his feet weeping, she began to wet his feet with her tears. Then she wiped them with her hair, kissed them and poured perfume on them.

[39] When the Pharisee who had invited him saw this, he said to himself, "If this man were a prophet, he would know who is touching him and what kind of woman she is – that she is a sinner."

[40] Jesus answered him, "Simon, I have something to tell you."

"Tell me, teacher," he said.

[41] "Two people owed money to a certain moneylender. One owed him five hundred denarii,[a] and the other fifty. [42] Neither of them had the money to pay him back, so he forgave the debts of both. Now which of them will love him more?"

[43] Simon replied, "I suppose the one who had the bigger debt forgiven."

"You have judged correctly," Jesus said.

[44] Then he turned toward the woman and said to Simon, "Do you see this woman? I came into your house. You did not give me any water for my feet, but she wet my feet with her tears and wiped them with her hair. [45] You did not give me a kiss, but this woman, from the time I entered, has not stopped kissing my feet. [46] You did not put oil on my head, but she has poured perfume on my feet. [47] Therefore, I tell you, her many sins have been forgiven – as her great love has shown. But whoever has been forgiven little loves little."

⁴⁸ *Then Jesus said to her, "Your sins are forgiven."*

⁴⁹ *The other guests began to say among themselves, "Who is this who even forgives sins?"*

⁵⁰ *Jesus said to the woman, "Your faith has saved you; go in peace."*

Regardless of the source we choose, it seems this particular Bible story is incomplete. To hear the beginning of the story we must go right back to eight days after the day of Christ's birth.

The **First Book of the Infancy of Christ** is a gospel that was given to the Gnostics, a Christian sect from the second century onwards. This particular book of the apocrypha was gained from Peter Martyr, Bishop of Alexandria, in the 3rd century.

In Chapter II we read:

AND when the time of his circumcision was come, namely, the eighth day, on which the law commanded the child to be circumcised, they circumcised him in the cave.

2 And the old Hebrew woman took the foreskin (others say she took the navel-string), and preserved it in an alabaster-box of old oil of spikenard.

3 And she had a son who was a druggist, to whom she said, Take heed thou sell not this alabaster box of spikenard-ointment, although thou shouldst be offered three hundred pence for it.

Now this is that alabaster-box which Mary the sinner procured, and poured forth the ointment out of it upon the head and the feet of our Lord Jesus Christ, and wiped it off with the hairs of her head.

So, here, opens up a whole new array of questions for me. Could there really be such a thing as the Holy Foreskin soaked in spikenard, in existence?

Famously, yes.

It appears that the *Holy Prepuce* became a relic of great consternation to the Church, because for a period of time they seemed to be popping up everywhere (If you will pardon the pun!).

The first appeared in AD800, when it was given to Pope Leo II by the Emperor Charlamagne when he had crowned him. Charlamagne explained that he had been given it by an angel as he prayed ,although other documentation suggests that he may have been given it by the Empress Irene as a wedding present. At one point there were thought to be 21 of these Holy Foreskins around the world, (even in Stoke on Trent, famously home to Take That!) The Christian world naturally flocked to see the relics because they were reputed to be part of His body. Powers were attributed to the relics, in particular that they may be able to protect women in childbirth.

One of the relics was housed in Charroux, France, which in the 16th century, suddenly started to drip drops of blood and Pope Clement III deemed that this was miraculous and so Charroux must have the real one.

Eventually in the 1900's the Church decided to distance itself from the controversy of the Holy Foreskin. They ruled it inappropriate to be giving so much attention to this intimate part of Christ's anatomy. It was announced that any other foreskin than that from Charroux must be a fraud and it was threatened that anyone speaking or writing about it would be excommunicated. So, I hope this particular part of spikenard's history does not injure my future too much!

A strange coincidence did surprise me though. A common medieval school of thought was that every one of the foreskins must be a fake, because theologians felt that it must have ascended into Heaven when Christ did. The point that gave me pause was that 17th century theologian Leo Allatius speculated in his essay *De Praeputio Domini Nostri Jesu Christi Diatriba* that the Holy Prepuce had risen and become the rings of Saturn. You'll see, later, that spikenard's ruling planet is none other than....

Saturn.

Is that or is that not mighty weird?

Spikenard at His Tomb

There are countless mentions on the internet of how spikenard was taken by Joseph of Arimathea to Christ's tomb, but this is inaccurate. Scripture tells us he took Oils of Myrrh and Aloeswood (what you and I would now recognise as Agarwood). There is, however, a rather controversial catholic document that suggests that spikenard may have played a part. The question is do we believe it?

Anne Catherine Emmerich was an Augustinian nun who lived 1774-1824 in Agnetenberg, Dulmen, Westphalia in Germany. Throughout her life she experienced many visions of the life and suffering of Jesus Christ, thought to have been shown to her by the Blesséd Virgin Mary. It is thought she had more visions than any other saint in history. Some were of the past, some the present and on rare occasions some were of the future. Her visions were very detailed and descriptive and when you read the treatise of her visions "The Dolorous

Passion of Our Lord Jesus Christ" it is hard to imagine that she was never there.

In 1802, Sister Emmerich began to show signs of the Crown of Thorns, in 1812, the full stigmata began. Her hands and feet bled and she developed a strange Y shaped mark over her breast bone. People who saw it felt certain they could see a cross over her heart and a wound from the lance.

By the end of 1818, the stigmata had stopped and whilst some were convinced of its authenticity, others considered her a fraud. In 1819 authorities took her away from her home and placed her in a separate house away from the other nuns. The visions continued.

In the later years of her life as she had become bedridden. Many doctors examined her but could find no cause for the marks. During the days of the stigmata, she was visited by a famous poet Clemens Bretano, who proceeded to write two works about her. The first was *The Dolorous Passion* (from which we will study a passage in a moment) which was to subsequently become the source material for Mel Gibson's banned film *The Passion of Christ*.

The Dolorous Passion is a difficult passage to study, because it is impossible to separate the thoughts of the nun from what have been described as "conscious elaborations of an overwrought romantic poet".

As modern day readers there is no denying the beautiful language is engaging and convincing but we can see a darker side that is nowhere near as nice. It casts a dark shadow over the text. Brentano's writings about Emmerich describe her as believing that Noah's son Ham was the progenitor of "the black, idolatrous, stupid nations" of the world. The "Dolorous Passion" also has a thinly veiled a "clear anti-Semitic strain throughout". Activists in the crucifixion of Christ are portrayed as being outrageously wicked and obsessed with chasing the Man to his death. There are assertions that the nun believed that "Jews ... strangled Christian children and used their blood for all sorts of suspicious and diabolical practices." In places we see her describing the Jews as *hook nosed* and other racist descriptions.

So then, we have to ask ourselves who thought these things? From a ghost writer's point of views (because as you know that is another part of my job) it is interesting to wonder where did her opinions stop and Bretanos begin? Did the bigotry belong to one or the other or is it a rather unpleasant combination of the two?

The second book *The Life of The Blessed Virgin Mary* was prepared in 1833, but Bretano died in '42. The book was eventually published posthumously in 1752.

Neither Bretano or Emmerich had ever visited Ephesus but in 1881, a French priest, the Abbé Julien Gouyet used the Sister's visions of The Blessed Virgin Mary to try to locate the virgin's house. The visions had also been used when the town was excavated and it is thought that it lead to the discovery of Mary's house prior to her Assumption.

In 1892, there were requests to the Vatican to consider Emmerich for beatification. Experts collated Bretano's writings and compared them to apocryphal writings, maps, and Biblical sources. Eventually in 1923 a German priest asserted that Bretano had fabricated most of the work and by 1928 an edict was made that only a very small part of the work could, in fact, be attributed to Emmerich. This assertion, though, was not released and instead the route to beatification was halted with no explanation to the outside world. In 1973 it was decided the case for her beatification could be reopened but only if Bretano's writings were set aside.

In 2003, it was decreed that there was a miracle about her and in 2004, Sister Anna Catherine Emmerich was beatified by Pope John Paul II, but the writings of Bretano were set aside.

The decision that Sister Emmerich could be prayed to, for requests of intercession, was based entirely on her unquestionable sanctity and virtue. Father Peter Gumpel had been one of the analysts in the decision as to whether to beatify the nun, even though some of the writings of the Dolorous Passion were questionable. He remarked *"Since it was impossible to distinguish what derives from Sister Emmerich and what is embroidery or additions, we could not take these writings as criteria. Therefore, they were simply discarded completely from all the work for the cause."* In 2006, Pope Benedict XVI visited the house which had been thought to be Mary's and treated it as a Holy Shrine.

So why are *we* interested in Sister Catherine? Well...

She talks of how spikenard was brought the tomb of Christ after his crucifixion, before the resurrection. I have used quite a full excerpt to give you a real feel for the haunting authenticity of her sight. But how much is Emmerich and how much Bretano?

Towards the close of the Sabbath-day, John came to see the holy women. He endeavoured to give some consolation, but could not restrain his own tears, and only remained a short time with them. They had likewise a short visit from Peter and James the Greater, after which they retired to their cells, and gave free vent to grief, sitting upon ashes, and veiling themselves even more closely.

The prayer of the Blessed Virgin was unceasing. She ever kept her eyes fixed interiorly on Jesus, and was perfectly consumed by her ardent desire of once more beholding him whom she loved with such inexpressible love. Suddenly an angel stood by her side, and bade her arise and go to the door of the dwelling of Nicodemus, for that the Lord was very near. The heart of the Blessed Virgin leaped for joy. She hastily wrapped her cloak about her, and left the holy women, without informing them where she was going. I saw her walk quickly to a small entrance which was cut in the town wall, the identical one through which she had entered when returning with her companions from the sepulchre.

It was about nine o'clock at night, and the Blessed Virgin had almost reached the entrance, when I saw her stop suddenly in a very solitary spot, and look upwards in an ecstasy of delight, for on the top of the town wall she beheld the soul of our Lord, resplendent with light, without the appearance of a wound, and surrounded by patriarchs. He descended towards her, turned to his companions, and presenting her to them, said, 'Behold Mary, behold my Mother.' He appeared to me to salute her with a kiss, and he then disappeared. The Blessed Virgin knelt down, and most reverently kissed the ground on which he had stood, and the impression of her hands and knees remained imprinted upon the stones. The sight filled her with *inexpressible joy, and she immediately rejoined the holy women, who were busily employed in preparing the perfumes and spices. She did not tell them what she had seen, but her firmness and strength of mind was restored. She was perfectly renovated, and therefore comforted all the rest, and endeavoured to strengthen their faith.*

All the holy women were sitting by a long table, the cover of which hung down to the floor, when Mary returned; bundles of herbs were heaped around them, and these they mixed together and arranged; small flasks, containing sweet unctions and water of spikenard, were standing near, as also bunches of natural flowers, among which I remarked one in particular, which was like a streaked iris or a lily. Magdalen, Mary the daughter of Cleophas, Salome, Johanna, and Mary Salome, had bought all these things in the town during the absence of Mary. Their intention was to go to the sepulchre before sunrise on the following day, in order to strew these flowers and perfumes over the body of their beloved Master.

I am not sure why I have decided to add this passage in really, except that it seems to have that same *is it? / isn't it?* vibration to it that the whole spikenard story seems to have. That, and the fact that legend has it, that the young nuns in her convent used to give her a wide berth because they found her incredible religious zeal, but paradoxical weak health, so very strange and unsettling. In her frail state there is nothing but certainly in her. Somehow that seems similar to the rest of the

Exodus story, Mary at the crucifixion and even our beautiful Phoenix.

If you would like to read more of her extraordinary meditations, including her detailed description of the chalice used at the Last Supper, you can find them at:

http://www.jesus-passion.com/DOLOROUS_PASSION_OF_OUR_LORD_JESUS_CHRIST.htm

The Revelation of St Peter

The *Revelation of Peter* is a 2nd Century early Christian document, probably written around 100AD. Whilst it is not in the New Testament, it is listed in the *Muratorian Fragment* which is the oldest surviving list of New Testament books which also stipulates that it must not be read in Church. An ancient Greek version was found by Sylvain Grébaut during the 1886-87 excavation of the necropolis at Akhmum in Upper Egypt. We think that the parchment had been placed into the grave of a 8th Century monk. Later in 1910, an Ethiopian version of the text was also found. In it the Apostles beg Jesus to show them what life will be like for them after death. Accordingly two angels stood before them:

"their bodies whiter than any snow and redder than any rose . . . and their shoulders like a wreath woven of spikenard and bright flowers, and their raiment so bright that they could not be looked upon."

Pope Francis and St Joseph:

Interestingly the current Pope has spikenard on his coat of arms. Because he is a Jesuit, at the top is the familiar name of Jesus IHS emblazoned in sunburst, there is an eight pointed star to signify Mary the mother of Jesus and beside it is a spikenard flower, designed to represent St Joseph.

St Joseph has always been pictured holding a spikenard flower in Hispanic iconography, but the reason and logic for it seems to have become lost in the annals of time. I wonder if it relates to Song of Songs and the obvious love for a virgin. After all, he was a bridegroom too. According to Matthew 1:25, he respected her chastity and never consummated the marriage. We spoke earlier of how the heiro gamos was a union of mortal and deity, with the spikenard being used as a crown of divinity. It seems only right that Joseph hold that sacred sign.

In a book of Spanish poetry, A Woman in Her Garden: Selected Poems, by Cuban, Dulce Maria Loynaz, is found this verse:

"Planted in your spell-bound earth, dry twigs turn to spikenard, white flower of Saint Joseph, the wedding flower."

Strangely, the common Spanish names for *Polianthes tuberosa*, our tuberose are *Nardo* or *Vara de San Jose* (Staff of St. Joseph). Some statues or pictures of St. Joseph depict him with a staff with a flower on top. Most of the time the ones toward the bottom are in bloom and those at the top are closed. Remember what Pliny said? There were 12 types of Nard, and one was tuberose? Perhaps we have had it wrong all a long! Tuberose certainly smells better in my opinion!

Chapter 4: A Treasure Of Its Time

Trade Routes

So, to me this seems extraordinary. This rather innocuous plant finds its way from the silence of the Himalayas across the world into pyramids, temples and the hullabaloo of parties and family celebrations. Regular readers will know I am rather captivated by the vision of the merchant and his caravan of camels so I wanted to understand the journey this medicine and perfume would have to take to get to its customers.

Archaeological evidence shows that there has been trading in spices since the 10th Millennium BC, however it was not actually documented until the Egyptians began to record trade in the 3rd Century BC. They traded spices in the Red Sea and across The Land of Punt.

In 2004, Delaware University revealed the findings of the port of Berenike, in Egypt. Romantically, this port had originally been founded by Ptolemy II (and named after his mother) in 265 BC, for the express intent of importing *elephants*! Recent relations with India had become so bad that India had cut off supply of the elephants that Ptolemy desperately needed to secure the lands of Seleucids to the North East. The natural harbour then, was a perfect, safe and protected place to bring

African elephants that Egyptians had captured into the country. This ancient trading post exposed the truth that goods from India had not only travelled across hot dry sands, that they had also travelled by sea.

Since excavations began in 1994, archaeologists have uncovered many papyri and ostraca (bits of pottery) that have shown wares arriving from a variety of countries. Amongst the evidence we find from south and southwest India came:

Nard, malabathron (a cinnamon ointment of antiquity), pepper, pearls, ivory, tortoise shell, transparent gems, diamonds, sapphires, silk cloth and cotton garments.

And from the Northeast:

Nard, malabathron, pearls, ivory and fine cotton garments.

Although not all scholars agree, there is strong evidence that this port at Berenike concentrated on importing *luxury* items destined to be traded throughout the Roman Mediterranean.

Robert James Forbes, in his *Studies in Ancient Technology*, reveals that in Corinthian, spikenard was used as eyepaint (This was because the Greeks felt that knitted eyebrows were a sign of great potency so men and women alike used to try to fake it by burning spikenard roots and then painting them on). He reveals that it was traded at Alexandria.

Muzaris was an ancient seaport and commercial centre on the Malabar Coast which we would now recognise as Kerala. (It is still not entirely clear where its exact location was. In 2006 there were claims that it had been found, but the fast announcement after its excavation promoted distrust and scepticism of the find.) Documents show it dating back to the 1st century BC or possibly before. It was a key trading post with the Phoenicians, Persians, Egyptians, Greeks and Romans. Commodities known to be traded from Muzaris were spices such as black pepper, pearls, diamonds, sapphires, ivory, silk, tortoise shells and Gangetic spikenard. In return the Romans brought in gold coins, copper, lead, thin linens, glass and wine.

Pliny suspected that the export of gold to India and China from the Roman Empire was just as much of a strain on the imperial resources as the large estates of slaves they were running. He estimated that 100 million sesterces a year were being exported to China, via India to pay for the silk trade. The entire luxury trade outside of the empire being calculated as much as 550 million sesterces. India was exporting goods to the Empire at 100 times their actual cost.

One consignment bound for Alexandria from Musaris contained 700-1,700 pounds of nard, 4700 lb Ivory, 790 lb textiles. The consignment was valued at 131 talents which would have been enough to purchase 2400 acres of the finest Egyptian farmland.

Don't imagine, either that this was one full ship. Oh no. The average Roman cargo ship held around 150 consignments of this size. The Romans, fully aware of the enormous prices they were being charged cynically encouraged the massive Indian trade, then levied 25% tax on all exports to the East at the Red Sea port of Lecce.

Roman trade dried up after the 5th century, but Musaris remained a commercial giant until the 14th century trading with the Persians, Arabs and Chinese.

The Periplus of the Erithraean Sea is a document of ancient Greek origin which relates trade routes of the period. Common opinion agrees it is probably 1st Century CE. It describes how nard was also exported from Barugaza (Bharoch) in the North and also Bareke near Beypore.

The translator of the Periplus was an American authority on antiquarian documents called Wilfred F Schoff, and interestingly enough he also wrote a monograph on "Nard" published in the The American Oriental Journal. In it he explains there might even be some problems with the translation of the word there too.

He explains than in a Roman digest of law between Marcus Aurelius and Commodus, Nard is listed as one of the items we spoke of earlier that were subject to duties into Egypt from the East.

Here, though, "Nard" and "The Spike of Nard" are classified separately. Nard is specified as the "Folium" that we have come to expect, but that then, has three further subdivisions.

- Pentasphaerum
- Barbaricum
- Caryophyllum

Pentasphaerum seems to relate to the balls and the leaf and fibre of the cinnamon laurel (or some identify it as betel pepper). In other documents, such as the Periplus, we see this listed as malabrathrum. This would mean that malabrathrum is yet another item to add to our ever growing list of things that nard can be!

Barbaricum refers to the point at the mouth of the Indus.

Caryophyllum means nut leaf and later was used as taxonomy to pertain to clove but also might mean the papery outside of a nutmeg that we know as mace.

However...again, these identifications might be dubious because cloves and mace are from the Archipelago of islands around Indonesia and of course Ptolemy mentions nard and fixatives as specifically being from the Himalayas. Neither is there proof that nutmegs had found their way to Greece by this period.

There are many Islamic writings from the Golden Age of the Caliphate (750-1150AD) about how liberally nard is received from the archipelago, but we do not find "True Nard" mentioned within then. For example, Ibn Khordadhbeh was the earliest Arabic geographical writer we have to refer to. His work the 9th Century *Kitab al-Masalik wa al-Mamalik* (*Of Roads and Realms*) is extremely important because it details commerce with the Jewish tribes in detail which is very unusual in his contemporaries. He says that Indian Nard is from Sumatra.

Twelfth century cartographer and geographer Al Idrisi says it is a product of Salahat.

Adu'l Fadl Jafar, in the Twelfth century cites Nard as being "idhkir", which says Schoff is most definitely a grass of the Andropogon family. In the 13th Century document Greek Muslim *Yāqūt ibn-'Abdullah al-Rūmī al-Hamawī* describes exports from Sumatra is being aloes, cloves, camphor, nard, mace, as well as drugs and vases from China.

Ibn al Baitar, Spanish botanist, philosopher and pharmacist from the 13th century was extremely interested in trade of specimens in particular and he speaks of three types of nard:

the *Sunbul*, which they call Indian Nard, in addition to Greek and Mountain Nard.

Then he tells us that Indian Nard is further classified into two sub species.

Sunbul At-tib

Sunbul al Asafir

I wonder, does this remind you of what Dioscorides had said? That there were two types of Nard – Indian and Syrian?

Later I shall show you some notes from the Twelfth Century Syriac Book of Medicines. It too distinguishes between two varieties. The translator AE Wallis Budge (same man who translated The Book of The Dead) equated the word *Nardin* with the Arabic sunbul.

Again, 13th Century Kazwini says that nard comes from Sumatra, Ceylon and the Islands of the East.

The point being of course that the True Nard can only come from India, so these others are patently another species/thing. I suspect that many of them are malabrathrum.

Economic Value

Earlier we saw the transcripts of the cargoes being moved along the Silk Route. Amongst the precious gems, our treasured Nard seemed to sit perfectly very happily, didn't it? So we must wonder just how pricey it was.

Pliny gives us an answer in his work, Natural History where he speaks extensively about the relative price comparisons between spices, resins and oils. This gives us a sparking insight into, not only the relative value of spikenard as a treasure, but also how it may have been used.

He estimated that Rome spent around 100 million sesterces per annum on incense from Arabia *alone*. It is still impossible to translate that into our money, but it is now known that 4 sesterces was the average daily wage (1 denarius was made up of 4 sesterces), which makes it seem an exorbitant amount of money.

Spikenard or nard oil was the most valuable of the oils and resins and could cost anywhere from 100, 75, to 40 denarii per pound depending on its quality (So by my reckoning even the rubbish stuff was going to cost you a month's wages – Agreed?).

In relation Myrrh was priced at anywhere from 3 to 50 denarii, and was often "*adulterated with pieces of mastic, and other gums; and drugged with the juice of wild cucumber*" (12.35.16). The finest frankincense could fetch a price of at 6 denarii per pound.

What's interesting too, is that figure, 100 denari for spikenard does not correlate with the price we see in the Bible. Could Mary have had a flask with 3lbs of ointment in? Probably not. More likely is we are seeing a demonstration of the massive fluctuation of value this antiquarian treasure could demand.

Spikenard in the Roman Kitchen

The Latin word for bitterness is *amaritudo* and the same word is used for *sharpness* and *heat of spices*. This was highly esteemed in the Roman kitchen. Cooks were liberal with their usage of herbs and spices.

According to Apicus the list of spices that one must have in the house "that nothing may be wanting" are:

Saffron, pepper, ginger, laser (?), aromatic leaves, myrtle berries, costmary, chervil, lemongrass, cardamom and spikenard.

Naturally foods, as today, were sorted with appropriateness to the time of year. Where I would make a beef stew in January, to warm the insides, according to Heirophilus the Sophist one should consume birds or fried fish seasoned with the hottest spices-pepper, cinnamon, spikenard or mustard. Roast suckling pig too, this time with a spiced gravy made from spikenard.

Those of robust constitutions may chose from a dry soup made of pepper, spikenard, cinnamon, cloves and the best storax, blended together with a small amount of honey. Alternatively, again, not for those with a sensitive tum, quince marmalade blended with a little lemon, pear, pomegranate, dates and cream mixed with spikenard. Stir into .durum wheat gruel. To wine, we are told "Your sweet wine should be spiced wine including pepper, spikenard and cloves." That's it! I am starting a renaissance. Let's get spikenard back into our kitchens!!!

A popular dish, again according to Andrew Dalby in his book *"The Flavours of Byzantium"* was Emmer Groats, an oats dish sweetened with spikenard. cinnamon and honey. (It sounds delish!)

Fenugreek seed was recommended by dieticians of the period, in three different ways, as a meal to be eaten in March. Consume it both as a seed and a sprouted seed as well as a soup. At all times sweeten it with cinnamon, honey and spikenard.

Pliny refers to a sweet spiced wine called Hypocras being made with spikenard. Sadly, I cannot find an original recipe. This one is from the 14th Century from the Menagier of Paris. Here a young wife of sixteen is given lessons in etiquette and housekeeping from her husband aged sixty! The book was written at the young woman's behest, with her acknowledging that she would be widowed young and the education might be well employed in her second marriage. Other books contemporaneous to the period replace galangal with spikenard.

To make a lot (=liquid measure) fine hippocras. Take one ounce cinnamon called long cinnamon in sticks, with some pieces of ginger and as much galanga, grind well together. Have a pound of fine sugar, and grind together and mix with a lot of the best wine of Beaune you can get and let this stand for one or two hours. Then let it run through a sack several times until it is clear.

Archaeological Evidence

We have documentary evidence aplenty. We have preponderances and discussions from scholars as to what their thoughts about what Nard might be. But where is the absolute categorical evidence that *Nardostachys jatamansi* was the plant the ancients were speaking of?

When I was writing the blog post about spikenard at Christmas, I came across an Egyptian page that sent me on a long and fascinating line of enquiry.

We read in Howard Carter's journal of the recovery of treasures from Tutankhamen's tomb on 22nd November 1922...

Our sensations and astonishment are difficult to describe as the better light revealed to us the marvellous collection of treasures: two strange ebony-black effigies of a King, gold sandalled, bearing staff and mace, loomed out from the cloak of darkness; gilded couches in strange forms, lion-headed, Hathor-headed, and beast infernal; exquisitely painted, inlaid, and ornamental caskets; flowers;

alabaster vases, some beautifully executed of lotus and papyrus device; strange black shrines with a gilded monster snake appearing from within; quite ordinary looking white chests; finely carved chairs; a golden inlaid throne; a heap of large curious white oviform boxes; beneath our very eyes, on the threshold, a lovely lotiform wishing-cup in translucent alabaster; stools of all shapes and design, of both common and rare materials; and, lastly a confusion of overturned parts of chariots glinting with gold, peering from amongst which was a manikin.

The first impression of which suggested the property-room of an opera-house of a vanished civilization. Our sensations were bewildering and full of strange emotion. We questioned one another as to the meaning of it all. Was it a tomb or merely a cache?

A sealed-doorway between the two sentinel statues proved there was more beyond, and with the numerous cartouches bearing the name of Tut-ankh-Amen on most of the objects before us, there was little doubt that there behind was the grave of that Pharaoh.

In that list of treasures lies a definitive line of enquiry that scholars had been waiting 2000 years to find. An alabaster vase...specifically "of lotus and papyrus device".

The diary tells us that the vase, later to become known by its artefact reference number 210, was not cleaned and inspected for another twelve months. His diary entries in February tell of how his colleague and he worked on the vases.

6th Feb

Commenced treating the cosmetic vase no. 211. It was badly stained by the fatty or oily substance it contained, which was still soft to a certain degree. Unfortunately it has eaten the aragonite in places, but by careful soaking in benzine I hope to get it in fair good order.

It is a very interesting and good piece of workmanship.

7 Feb.

Completed the aragonite cosmetic jar no. 211. I found that after removing as much of the stains as possible it was better to paraffin wax it. Now that it is cleaned it shows up admirably and is an exquisite example of design. Especially the heads of the captives upon which it stands - two negroes and two northerners of Mediterranean type.

Dr Munthe paid us a visit and lunched with us in the Valley.

Commenced experimenting on the large calcite vase 210, with caryatid figures - Nile gods HAPI. The problem here is how best to dissolve the content which has caused the frail neck to burst in many pieces.

Other contemporaneous records to the work, presumably belonging to the colleague he mentions, detail how the contents seemed to smell like valerian. Chemical analysis at the time showed that the unguent was mainly animal fats with some balsam and some vegetable oils that at the time were impossible to identify.

Before we move on, I thought you might like to read some of the extracts about opening the mummy and the details he wrote about his embalming discovery. (Note the date. He's brave unwrapping a mummy...!)

"October 31

All the moveable objects upon the exterior of the mummy were removed today.

I then attempted to remove the mummy and mask from the coffin, but found that unfortunately both were stuck fast to the bottom of the coffin, and could not be under the present conditions raised out without using great force, such as would endanger both the royal remains and the finely wrought mask.

The libation that was poured over the body had consolidated at the bottom and stuck them fast. My one hope now is that the heat of the sun may soften it sufficiently so as to enable one to gradually loosen mummy free it and raise it. If not, unless some other expedient is discovered, we shall have to make the examination as it lies within the two coffins.

With regard to the libation It would appear from the material that this substance it is composed of - seemingly fatty or oily substance mixed with (?) wood-pitch - that it is more an ointment than a libation. This oil liquid or ointment no doubt was applied in religious ceremony for the consecration of the dead king before appearing before the Great God (Osiris) of the underworld. It is particularly noticeable that on both the third coffin and the mummy the head and feet have been carefully avoided, even though the feet of the first coffin were anointed with a similar material.

Remark the episode that occurred "in the house of Simon the leper" when "there came a woman having an alabaster box of ointment of spikenard very precious; ... she is come aforehand to anoint my body to the burying." Mark 14, 1-8.

He too, seems to be thinking about the strange alabaster box.

If you would like to read more of Carters diaries about his remarkable excavation, you can find them at:

http://www.griffith.ox.ac.uk/discoveringTut/journals-and-diaries/season-1/journal.html

More recently, internet lore tells us that the principal ingredient in the "Unguent Vase with Magnificent Symbols" was in fact...Nardostachys jatamansi, although try as I might I could not find the paper that proved this. So I contacted Dr Lise Manniche, Egyptologist and author of one of my favourite books *Sacred Luxuries*. She, neither, could recall any papers confirming that spikenard had been confirmed as being in Tut's tomb, so personally I remain unconvinced. However, it may be so.

In fact, I have scoured so much archaeological data to try to find a definitive clue, I have nearly gone mad. Perfumery shops were found intact at Pompeii, Herculaneum and on the Greek island of Delos. Vials were also found on a shipwreck in St Gervais. Analyses of the Pompeii finds are that they contained "olive based perfumes". Flagons from the tombs of Valadas and the Roman necropolis at Saint Paul Trois Chateau contained "animal and vegetable fats". Unguentarii found at a necropolis in Lyon had, not just animal and vegetal fats, but also vegetal gums, and the experts surmised that rather than being a perfume, this might have been some kind of medicine.

In every case though the outcome was the same, that the volatile components had vanished and that chemical analyses on finds like these are far too few to be able to make comparisons in order to understand exactly what the ingredients may have been.

But then I finally made a breakthrough. The details of chemical analysis of thirty nine *unguentaria* (the name which is given to the alabaster amphorae containing unguents) from around 100BC to early Roman times which are housed in the Milwalkee Public Museum. Jenna Mortenson was able confirm very close matches between the main ingredient in the remains and our *Nardostachys jatamansi* of today, thus proving that the plant we now recognise as spikenard was used in Biblical times. Whilst it is not completely the Nard of the Ancients, because we now recognise Nardostachys to be merely an ingredient of the product *Nard* which was a concocted perfume, it brings us a little closer to understanding what it might have been. It remains to be proven that it spikenard was in Mary's alabaster box, though, since as we know nard could have been any number of things.

Somehow though, the uncertainty seems correct here. Spikenard in its ethereal majesty winks and says...you just can't be sure can you. You'll just have to have a little faith won't you?

And perhaps....that's just how the Great Creator likes it.

Mortenson's findings from the ungentaria can be found here: http://dc.uwm.edu/cgi/viewcontent.cgi?article=1511&context=etd

Part 2: Nardostachys jatamansi

Ayurvedic Medicine

Just as a recap, because my head is swimming with what is, what isn't and what may be. Nardostachys maybe (almost certainly is) the Spikenard of the Ancients. It *is* the spikenard we use in aromatherapy and it *is* the plant which is so highly acclaimed in Ayurveda.

It is considered to be divine and is used as an air purifier ready for the act of prayer. It is used as part of pooja, daily prayers, but also specifically during the ritual of yagna.

Performed in front of the sacred fire, agni, incenses are sprinkled on to send messages of sacrifice in this mighty act of devotion to the gods. As the spikenard fragrance fills the air, mantras are chanted in reverence to spirit.

Spikenard is one of the most esteemed of all the Ayurvedic medicines, because it enhances the body's ability to sleep and thus repair.

It balances and coordinate **Prana Vata** (governs **the mind**) and **Sadhaka Pitta** (governs **the emotions**). Its long term effect influences **Tarpaka Kapha** that coordinates the laws of nature governing health of the **sinus cavities, head and cerebral-spinal fluids**. This acts to stabilize the emotions. The *Chakara*

Samhita recommends it highly for **insomnia**, for **mental instability** and to **enhance memory.**

The next one you are going to ẅant underline...

It is said to promote growth and maintain the colour of hair.

It is a **strong sedative** and since it is a close relative of valerian it exerts the same relaxing qualities **to over stimulated minds.**

It is very useful in calming **hyperactive children.**

In Ayurveda they use the whole plant, but the root and rhizomes, which is what the essential oil is distilled from, ar given for **hysteria, heart palpitations, menopause** and **nervous diseases.**

Now, if this is the first of my essential oils profiles that you have read, you may need to take in a bit of background into the doshas before you move forward. To prevent repletion I have hidden this for you at the back of the book. Read a <u>Brief Introduction to Ayurveda</u> (Page 371) before reading on, or I may as well be speaking Welsh to you!

Now, spikenard is such fascinating medicine because it is **cooling viriya** and **pungent vipaka** which means in some cases it will cool but in others, particular for digestive medicine, it will warm.

Actually vipaka means *post*-digestive, and that is 6-8 hours post digestive, so the effects come some hours after use. How does it do this? Well, Nardostachys enters into the rakta and majja dhatus.

The dhatua are the tissues of the body and there are seven of them. These are:

1. Plasma (Rasa)

2. Blood (Rakta)

3. Muscle (Mamsa)

4. Fat (Meda)

5. Bone (Asthi)

6. Bone marrow and nerve (Majja)

7. Reproductive fluid (Shukra)

The rakta dhatu refers to the primary fire of the body. It means reddened and coloured, but also impassioned. Physically it means the red blood cells of the body and indirectly to the tendons and bile. More though, than blood, it is the internal fire that invigorates the body and mind.

Close your eyes for a second and just repeat that to yourself, because I think it wholly sums up the medicine in the entirety.

Spikenard activates the internal fire that invigorates the body and mind

If raka dhatu is deficient then the body is cold and stiff but also the mind becomes sluggish and loses focus too.

Use spikenard...

Raktu dhatu is formed of the same qualities as fire. It is hot, dry and hard, unstable, tough. It flows and is clearing. It is both subtle *and* sharp. Thus spikenard also mimics these qualities.

It has a very special relationship with the liver. The liver forms the both source and the channel of this energy through which unstable rasa (plasma) must pass. (Well look at this in more detail in a moment.)

When rakhta dhatu becomes overheated so does rasa, as a result of this the liver and spleen, also becomes overheated and possibly enlarged. We see this, for example in hepatitis.

Use spikenard...

You might recognise these qualities as being similar to that of pitta dosha, when rakta dhatu depletes, so then does pitta dosha too. The person feels cold the skin becomes pale and lacks lustre. Coldness causes the body to hold onto sweat, in cases it loses any more heat and urination depletes too, followed them by constipation.

Using spikenard then, acts as a laxative and relieves the bladder. It restores a glow to the complexion, warming it by invigorating rakhta dhatu.

In this chilled mental and physical state the mind is too busy shivering to take in any new information. Processing becomes confused and forgetful. Misunderstandings and arguments begin to raise their troublesome heads.

Warming the mind, spikenard opens closed channels of thought and aids memory.

So that's when the energy in the channel is low but as we know the pendulum always swings both ways. Let's nudge it to see what rakta dhatu might look like in excess.

The body feels too warms and it looks for ways to release heat. Blood rushes to the capillaries in the surface of the skin and this vasodilation reddens the skin. There is an increase in urination and also stools become looser too. Sweating becomes problematic too.

Spikenard cools the body and eases the excretory process. Urge incontinence is reduced, diarrhoea is slowed and the redness in the skin subsides.

If the body cannot lose enough heat, then the inflammation spreads to the mucous membranes followed by the liver, there after each and every organ may be affected in turn.

Ok, turn the mirror and let's see it reflected from the point of pitta dosha.

Pitta dosha *increases* the fire of rakta dhatu. This increase means that you feel warmer and more emotionally intense.

So what can raise this?

- Intellectual study (too much)
- Too much exercise
- Food that is too hot and spicy

Eventually the body will burn out the dhatu. It can no longer hold onto the heat and it becomes cold and easily fatigued. Interestingly, it can be very easy for the inexperienced to see this as vata imbalance. It's not. It is <u>**burnout.**</u>

So when rakta dhatu increases, every bodily function becomes more intense. Periods, in particular, become very heavy and painful. The flow is very heavy, but only lasts for a couple of days.

Emotionally small things become very important, and troubling. One's sense of dharma seems to disappear.

(Dharma is one of those strange words that doesn't seem to have a translation. The closest I can come is the nourishment and fulfilment you get from something), the end result completely supersedes the processes one goes through to make something beautiful...thus creativity is crushed.

Physically, excess shows itself in the joints, in skin inflammations, redness of the eyes and sharply visible blood vessels.

You will usually find rheumatic disorders and also problems with connective tissues, or conversely you might see auto-immune responses that generate inflammation.

The two, rakta dhatu and pitta dosha are entirely inseparable, they are quintessentially linked to each other's health.

I also mentioned that jatamansi heated the body through *majja dhatu.*

Majja means *bone marrow*, however it has become synonymous with the *nervous system* because, like the bone marrow, this *system is encased within bone.* Think of the brain protected by the skull and the spinal cord housed within the vertebrae. In Ayurveda, bone marrow and the nervous systems, residing in the bone spaces, are treated as one system, majja. This is considered to be the sixth tissue of the body. Now, as we know, the nervous system is particularly wondrous because it reacts to signals that it receives both internally and externally. It transmits these to the brain, processes them and then reacts to them.

Majja has four main functions

- To nourish the bones
- Provide body strength
- Oversee brain and nervous system duties
- Responsible for mental and emotional states

The doshas of the body (vata, pitta, kapha) move from one part of the body to another through channels called srotami (or the singular of that plural is srotas). The largest channel is *Maha* (meaning largest) and that is the digestive tract, but inversely there are also teeny tiny srotami, single cells in the body only seen under a microscope. When you observe them magnified, you can see that they are porous. Srotamsi oxygen and nutrients can be absorbed through these channels and likewise CO_2 and waste products can be transported out too. Srotami then, act like pathways or roads *transporting information, nutrients and waste from one place to another*.

The srotami spikenard acts upon are:

- *Rasavara:* This runs from the right chamber of the heart and the ten great vessels. It rises at the venous and lymphatic systems and the capillaries.

- *Raktavaha* which acts as you might imagine on the liver and spleen. It tones the arteriole circulatory system and the venous junctions.

- *Anavaha-* This is the genitourinary tract

- *Majjavaha* – Again space between the bones, brain, spinal cord, but also the sympathetic and parasympathetic nervous system and the synaptic space (That's the space between the electrical impulses that trigger nerve messages)

- *Pranavaha* - Respiratory tract, nose and bronchial tree

- *Sukhravaha* – testicles and nipples, vas deferens (the tube that carries sperm out), urethra, prostate and GUI tract, in particular the urethral opening.

Spikenard then is used for its *antispasmodic* and *carminative* effects in these areas.

Actions
- *Medhya* (Brain tonic),
- *Rasayana* (Rejuvenative to the mind),
- *Nidhrajnana* (Promotes sleep),
- *Manasrogaghna* (Alleviates mental diseases),

- *Pachana* (Digestive),
- *Kasawasahara* (Alleviates - coughs and breathing difficulties),
- *Kushtaghna* (Stops skin diseases and itching),
- *Dahaprasha*- mana (Stops burning sensations),
- *Varnya* (Benefits complexion) and
- *Roma sanjanana* (Promotes - hair growth).

Usage

- Digestive esp. Flatulence
- Hyper-cholesterol
- Palpitations
- Effects of nervous upset
- Somatisation (Physical illness with no obvious physical cause)
- Jaundice
- Kidney Stones
- Respiratory Diseases
- Skin Diseases
- Typhoid
- Seminal debility
- Spasmodic hysterical states
- Epilepsy
- Convulsions

- Tension headaches
- Insomnia
- ADHD
- Febrile delirium
- Senile dementia
- Analgesic
- Anti-arrhythmic
- Hypotensive
- Promoter of hair growth

And in the same paradox as being **cooling** and **warming,** spikenard is both **stimulant** and **sedative**. This would be the primary reason for choosing for spikenard over valerian which dulls the senses.

Ethnobotany
A list of local traditional medical usages as found by the CITES survey taken as an aid to devising conservation plans.

India:

- Antispasmodic
- Stimulant
- Treatment of fits
- Heart palpitations
- Regulation of constipation,

- Regulation of urination,
- Menstruation
- Digestion

Nepal:

Used as:

- brain tonic
- uterine tonics
- stimulants,
- External pain killers,
- Antiseptic,
- Treatment of epilepsy,
- Hysteria,
- Convulsions,
- Heart palpitations,
- High blood pressure,
- Fever,
- Anxiety,
- Insomnia,
- Asthma and other bronchial problems
- Acidity

Used in the Dolpa region, rhizomes are used by *amchi* (traditional medicine practitioners trained in Tibetan medicine) for treating complaints including:

- Epilepsy,
- Wounds,
- Coughs,
- Colds
- High blood pressure

The Newar people of Katmandu burn the rhizomes in funeral rituals. In the Menang district of Nepal it is most beloved because when growing wild, it stays away from civilisation and so cannot be contaminated. Historically it has been burned in the Shikkim Himalayas as a protectorate, the smoke being reputed to scare away evil spirits.

In Nepal, it is used in tonics, stimulants, as an antiseptic, for the treatment of epilepsy, hysteria, convulsions and heart palpitations (Anon., 1993).

In Bhutan, it is used primarily as incense, mixed with other plants and burned in religious rites and ceremonies. It is. A very small quantity is used as an ingredient in the preparation of their indigenous medicine.

In China, the species is listed in the current version of the Pharmacopoeia of People's Republic of China (Anon., 1995a). Its use was first recorded in *The Compendium of Materia Medica,* compiled in the sixteenth century. According to literature on traditional Chinese medicine, spikenard is:

- Effective in pain relief,
- Regulating Qi,
- Treating a turgid chest (bronchial congestion)

Despite that the CITES survey revealed that N. grandiflora is not considered to be a commonly used medicinal plant in China.

In Pakistan, the species is collected to treat

- Hysteria
- Epilepsy
- Neurosis
- Insomnia
- Excitation
- Habitual constipation
- Scorpion stings

Under the name of *Asaroon*, the plant is used in nine herbal preparations, according to the Hamdard Pharmacopoeia, (*Qarabadain-eHamdard*), for treatment of

Hemiplegia, (paralysis down one side of the body

- Bell's Palsy,
- Parkinson's Syndrome,
- Tremors,
- Indigestion
- Deafness due to age.

They also use essential oil as a flavouring agent as well a cosmetic and perfume

.

Part 3 The Spiritual Aspects of Spikenard

We understand the physical side of the plant well now, and to an extent the emotional one. But every plant has a psychological aspect connecting our life lessons to the cosmos around us. To a great extent, this enables us to comprehend how spiritual challenges and crises can emanate into the physical body and in turn how, although we cannot exactly predict the future, we are able to determine how a plant might alter the pathway of a disease.

Ruling Planet

No-one who has used spikenard will be surprised that it is ruled by Saturn, the planet of trials and adversity, because most assuredly spikenard does make you feel like you can overcome any obstacle. When I write that, I worry one might get the vibration of a vitamin fuelled frenzy to take on the day. Actually what I mean is that calmness and resolve one needs as we stand at the foot of Everest, and decide that we will see the summit. It is calm, determined and in the clear cold atmosphere...it is very, very quiet.

Spikenard holds your hand gently and encourages you to gingerly take another look at that which seemed terrifying, and with the aroma of your grounding friend in your nostrils you can say, Ok, I can do this.

I have noticed that often people comment that they find this part of the book distracting because it feels too metaphysical for them so I thought I would put it into context. As we have gone through the history of how the ancients used the plant, we must ask ourselves how they came upon their wisdom, not least because, when we are testing their theories, two maybe three thousand years later, we find that for the most part they were correct and that's amazing. So how did that happen?

Most certainly there will have been trial and error, and they will have noticed trends of people healing (and dying, of course) after using certain herbs, but most of their ideas come from which ruling planet a plant was placed under. It will dictate which organs it helps, what kind of personalities (because that was oft discerned as part of their illness) and what emotions. These metaphysical parts of these Secret Healer books are not *my* ideas they are merely another translation of how a plant had been used before. To my own mind however, these ruling planets give us far more insights into the nuances of healing than a list of uses and actions in modern day text book ever could.

Let's do this a bit differently then. Ptolemy – the man who gave Sir William the clues that Nard might be a Valerian, would tell you that music and astronomy were inextricably linked so let's introduce you to the Saturnic landscape through Gustav Holst's Saturn from The Planet Suite.

Have a listen. Close your eyes and hear what the music tells you about the planet. Note every feeling you have about the piece and then we'll move on. https://www.youtube.com/watch?v=Qb79SiZrzvw

OK what does *Saturn* do then? In short, it tests our boundaries of personal experience. It makes life hard and relentless. Thus when we see a Saturnic lesson, we should think of spikenard as an antidote or at least a way of navigating its still, frozen landscape.

Did you find the music menacing at all? Rhythmic, bordering on predictable in places? Beautiful, but a bit boring at times, right? Did you have to turn it down because it got too much at any point? In fact, did you manage to get all the way through it without thinking "Enough already!"?

Saturn medicine puts us under pressure, restricting us in order that we might build much firmer foundations for the future. It shows us our perceptions of the finite limits of our capabilities are merely illusions and demonstrates that these are far more elastic than we thought. If we reach inside of ourselves, which Saturn will ensure that we do, or we simply won't survive, then we will see we are so much more than we imagined. It turns the screw tighter and tighter, upping the pressure and then upping it again. Its pitches itself against our willpower, and when we scream we've had enough, it simply jeers "Is that all you've got? You're going to need a whole lot more than that."

Saturn makes you tough.

Its influences insist you make the most of the resources available (inherent or material) and it demands that you create something stronger, bigger and better. And spikenard says, "Don't be afraid. I've got your back. Face it. Because I refuse to let you turn back."

(Regular readers might want to compare that with the hot and spicy pep talks from Sweet Basil which empowers you though heat and damn near shoves you into new situations, spikenard says: *Be cool.* We can take this as carefully as you like"

You need that too, because Saturn illuminates every limit of your fears, and forces you right up against them. It will spotlight self doubt. Any weakness or Achilles heel, Saturn will find it and demand that you man up and face it. And with spikenard you can, with far less pain than you would imagine.

(Interestingly, if you look at your birth chart, the house that Saturn occupies will also give you an indication of where your biggest insecurities lie. These are most likely the karmic lessons you were sent here to learn. That house where Saturn transited the moment you were born will always be your Achilles heel.)

It's interesting because where most of the planets energies are about moving forward on a spiritual journey and about higher learning, Saturn says "Hang on. Let's get real here!" He is *all* about reality, and that is very much a root medicine quality. (And here you can read medicines made from roots like vetiver and ginger, but also ones that affect the root chakra. That would also be true.) In fact, Saturn says let's make firmer foundations, get your feet back on the ground, let's really dig your roots more firmly into the earth. A Saturn lesson says "Where's your common sense, woman?" It will make you dig deep, get practical, pragmatic and canny.

If you have Saturn transiting through your second house in your astrological chart, the one that rules money, then money will be very tight. The benefit of that, of course, is when it leaves and moves into your third house, you have learned to live in next to nothing. You have become an Ebay expert, you know where all the bargains are to be found and you are coupon queen, so when the money starts to flow again, your finances are leaner and cleaner. Saturn feels like a right f**ker when he is staring at you but at the end you have always learned an extraordinary amount about yourself. More than that, you have found new safer land to settle than you were on before.

Saturn is the slowest moving planet in the solar system, taking between 29-30 years to do a full circuit. It is also very dim and unimpressive to view. So, it medical astrology, it has come to mean old age or simply a lack of vitality. It is careful, slow, determined. Likewise, as Saturn affects our borders, so it affects the "borders" of our body, our skin, teeth, hair and bones.

It is a cold planet. Unlike Mars, for instance, Saturn energy has no heat or fire. Likewise there is no passion or inflamed desire. Any movement is slow, deliberate and predictable. (Remember how it makes you feel like you might fall?) Depending on who you are, like me for instance, you might find that predictability reassuring, it might make others stir crazy and they might fin it terribly mundane.

For a moment, weigh your heart against that statement. If shocks and horrors have become too much, the spikenard will most assuredly be your friend. If you want something more exciting, then, a mars or Jupiter ruled medicine might be a better answer.

Traditional astrological texts refer to Saturn as "The Greater Malefic". Strangely for us, this term was first coined by our friend Ptolemy whom was the centre of the identification argument. As well as being a wonderful naturalist, Ptolemy had a deep interest in astrology and wrote what was to be the most scientific argument for the reasoning behind astrology, *The Tetrabilis*. Working from his observatory, Ptolemy catalogued a massive 700 stars, of which 300 were new discoveries! To understand the context of Ptolemy's theories, one must remember that in the second century, Saturn was the furthest planet, discovered, away from the sun. (Uranus was discovered 1781 and Pluto 1930.)

So, the Malefics represent **damage and loss**. Saturn is the greater, Mars being termed "Lesser malefic". They are extreme planets. Mars being far too hot and dry and Saturn being *cold* and dry. Since Saturn is so far away from the sun, he cannot be affected by her creative warmth. Likewise, he is too far away from Earth's moisture too. Therefore anything affected by Saturn's energy will eventually decay. Saturn then, becomes the ultimate agent of destruction and death.

It follows then that when there is a Saturn influence in your life, there can be no growth. Not yet anyway. We need to wait patiently for spring. This is a time of hibernation, of squirreling away and using resources very carefully indeed. The energy surrounding you is dark and utterly incapable of receiving any luminosity or generosity in life, thus you only have yourself to rely upon.

This absence of light also means that life feels heavy, of course. Life never feels very sure footed and there is more of a propensity to fall. In all, life feels weighed down, grave and sombre.

In short, when Saturn affects you, life gets very serious.

Heavy, man...

In terms of understanding spikenard medicine too, it's useful to envisage the sorts of places that Saturn rules over. Think of the terms "Cold", "Oppressive", "Restrictive". What sorts of places come to mind?

Prisons? Mental Health units? Old People's homes?

Yup, you got it. You might also think of things that govern decay and weakness, or anything that is representative of hard physical labour.

It's the sound of the man working on the chain gang. Guess what planet represents the shackles?!

https://www.youtube.com/watch?v=f5lYNgCVwFos

Since Saturn is in opposition to the sun, ancient seers would also call him Lord of Winter, the enemy of the sun. Remember how, when we have thought of Jupiter before (in the Holy Basil book) it was an authority, but in a nice way? He was justice? Well. Saturn, not so much. He is authoritarian all right, but this time like an over-zealous father who is far more interested in structure and process than happiness or obedience. So we might think of the oppression of the Hebrews in Egypt. We might think of the Jews under Roman (or, I suppose, also Pharisaic) rule. We might think of the plight of the Jews under Hitler. Terrible atrocities under *oppression*. Saturn was influencing and spikenard was there and we need to hold that "oppression" theme clearly in our minds.

Saturn has a "Because I said so" energy to it and there is always going to be a dimension where you think "What the hell's the point of fighting, I might as well just get on and do what he says, whether I like it or not".

It's all good, ayn it?

But spikenard says, "c'mon, no point complaining. Let's just get on with it.

Go with the flow.

And if you think Saturn sounds like a bit of a barstool, well, I am afraid, it only gets worse, because in order to learn Saturn's lessons (and there is no way that you can assimilate Uranus and Neptune gifts until you do), he demands some kind of sacrifice.

(Looks like we are into dried goat blood land again!)

There will be loss, but it is likely to be denial and *self* sacrifice rather than an actual goat!! In some dimensions we might think of him as the grim reaper, slashing away at our hopes and dreams, but we can also choose to see him as Father Time. This is planet that ensures we plan for the future, for he is in it for the long game.

Often Saturn will be connected in some way to our past and our history (think of how we have wasted money, for instance) but the lesson is often about *rehabilitation*. (Of offenders or psychiatric patients, but also just on an everyday basis of quit that ridiculous Starbucks habit...it is costing you hundreds of dollars a year, or another example maybe putting rocky relationships into separation, enforced or otherwise).

Saturn is always about the future...*Goddamn, boring astrological accountant.*

I am making light, but my own experiences of Saturn have been Darrell and I both losing our jobs in the same month, and then someone I love very dearly having to be sectioned because they had quite literally lost their mind.

It ain't nice.

But, if you see Saturn depicted in ancient writings, it is shown as a serpent, in a ring, eating its own tail (*now that's what I call sacrifice!*) So there is always this idea of regeneration, but also Saturn is the planet of karma, so we think of lessons not only for this life but also the next. Those, that if we refuse to get our heads down into the books and really learn, will come back and bite us in the asp again!

Asp....do we think venom? No, we think constrictor. So, just as Jupiter is expansion, then Saturn is constraint. We are going to see loss, failure and then all the emotional pain that ensues. Often the lesson is bloody hard, and you can't even perceive what the blasted lesson is...until the time has passed but then it will be clear.

Most certainly too, the lesson is beneficial. It's like getting double detention, really, I suppose! It brings about steadiness, stability and the long term investment always comes with rewards. It's quite an interesting project to discover where Saturn is in your chart right now, and to suss out what area he is affecting. Then think back 29 years, he would have been affecting the same things. When Saturn bashed my family last year, I cast my mind back and the same lesson was at work in entirely different ways. Both times I had had to learn new ways to relating to my parents.

If you can start to track these patterns, you will be able to discern the sacrifices made from your life each time. Then, you will always notice that these were reasoned and well thought out and completely fitting. Actually, you will find those things you shed, were dead already. They were neither use nor ornament and the time has long since passed when you should have shown them the door. This is the beauty of Saturn's winter pruning. What grows in the spring is always better.

Think of Saturn's cycle as a clock. The first cycle of a child's life looks like this.

At the first quarter, at 7 years old, he loses his baby teeth. At fourteen, then he enters puberty. At 21 he enters adulthood and a 29-30 you will often see some sort of loss. (Mine was an ectopic pregnancy.) Astrologers will tell you that there is no sense of maturity until a person has gone through that first "Saturn return" around your thirtieth birthday.

Often Saturn's winter coincides with feelings of loneliness and isolation – or maybe it might be better to say feeling like you are on your own. Either way, we will likely feel bereft. Perhaps there might be the loss of a business or simply of an idea, rather than a relationship of financial loss. Whatever the sacrifice is, this is Saturn's wake up call to face reality. Slap in the face it might be, but at least you can see things a lot more clearly.

Often as Saturn passes on, we do feel a little older, but in the good sense. We have a sense of slowing, of resting. We feel a kind of maturity from this wealth of valued experience. Then too, we might find we are happy to give up dreams and ambitions that we had been holding on to so tightly. There are a new set to be enjoyed. In order to benefit from Saturn's lesson, it requires that we go within, listen and really bear witness to what is happening around us. That's terrifying when you feel you are drowning in quicksand, but somehow spikenard moves you to the quietness at the eye of the storm and lets you quietly plan your next move.

Ruling Sign

Since it has Saturn rulership, then Spikenard is ruled by two signs: Capricorn and Aquarius. In Capricorn he is nocturnal and diurnal in Aquarius, and you can almost see these as the day and night qualities because Saturn is much more expressive in Aquarius.

Again Cap/Aqu corresponds to winter. To the cold. To hibernation. So in particular we see Capricorn connected with the elderly and the weak. I was interested to find it also rules the metal lead, because of its dull surface and the thick heavy sound it makes when it is bashed. Given Spikenard's close affiliation with anointing, it is also strange to recall that tombs are traditionally made of lead!

Incidentally, did you know two that the old fashioned name for lead poisoning is...*Saturnalia*? The symptoms of this illness are fatigue, depression, melancholy and a slowing down of mental processes. (Hang on, aren't those treated with spikenard?!)

People who have a lot of Capricorn in their chart tend to be quite austere. If you think of the zodiac as life, and that the first sign, Aries would be the baby...then these people would be the middle aged grownups. They are sensible and have enough strength left to enjoy their wisdom. Get that vibration and you are starting to feel spikenard's medicine.

These people think hard before they speak and as such then, when they do speak their words have weight. (A useful vibration to be able to summon up by a plant if you have a situation where you need to learn to keep your gob shut.) These are serious people. They have very profound imaginations, they can think magical and fantastical things but their *outward* acts in life are severe. They are very patient in their work and are happy with duties that the rest of us might consider to be toil.

They are studious and are drawn very deeply into anything that they do. These are deep, sincere and respected people.

They have a very deep sense of responsibility in life. Their emotions are well hidden, very deep, and they won't show them easily to people.

Are they plodders?

No, I don't think so. More, detached, accepting of their lot and feeling grateful for their place in life.

It is a really nice energy to be able to use spikenard to summon.

They are funny too, because these Capricorn/Aquarian people have the driest senses of humour there is. You won't even notice the giggle because they just do not crack their faces.

So, spikenard has this to say, in such a manner.

Always Look on The Bright Side Of Life:

Monty Python

https://www.youtube.com/watch?v=jHPOzQzk9Qoo,

 Mary's spikenard seemed to spread right over the hill, there, didn't it? Probably wholly inappropriate given some of the content about death later in the book, but in my defence...

It was the spikenard what made me do it, guv!

Of course, there is a negative side to these people too. That pendulum always swings equally both ways...

If the pendulum does swing, they are cynical and pessimistic. They can be very negative, suspicious and jealous. They will always feel like they are always living in the most hostile world. They lack trust and will sneer at anything that cannot be tested. (Naturally, it is going to be very hard to get these people to try any plant essence, let alone some Nard of The Ancients if you feel they require therapy!)

These people are materialistic, results driven, and this focus on the physical rather than emotional and spiritual elements of life can often jeopardise their relationships. The problem for them is almost the same as for the positive aspects, their feelings are *too* well hidden and so they have no comprehension if how to express them. Consequently, these repressed emotions will most likely develop into some kind of personality disorder....and we are round to spikenard again.

So, themes then....

And it helps I think to understand the theme rather than try to put it into context because you might just think the person is that theme or is suffering at the hands of it, and so then spikenard would be their prescribed medicine

- Authority
- Discipline
- Hard work
- Labour
- Commitment
- Guilt
- Resistance

- Duty
- Delay

Is the patient too authoritarian? Are they struggling under the heavy glare of an authoritarian parent? Is the wife left at home because the authoritarian state has locked her husband up? Authoritarian (or I suppose oppression, might be a better word) is a theme. It's not, however, necessarily a symptom, as such.

Think back to Holst again (or listen to it). Recall that bang, bang, bang, repetitive, almost droning cadence all the way through. This is very much Saturnic medicine feature. Boring, boring, boring, learn it again, and again, and again and again. Think of it a bit like weight training through resistance. It is discipline and practice that make you better, until it becomes an ingrained habit. You are more careful with money, you don't feel the need to be with the abusive partner, the business partnership breaks down and you learn to go it alone...And that there, is the essence of it. It does make you feel unloved and neglected and so you go off on your own and then...you grow into someone far more self sufficient.

Out Here On My Own:
Irene Cara

☐

https://www.youtube.com/watch?v=i4mkRwkQRoQ

And amongst all this cold, hard change it is difficult to hold on to anything positive and that is when you are at your most vulnerable to being emotionally sucked under. Spikenard steps in and says "Hold on. Hold on to that vision you had. You are strong enough and you can get through this to a much happier place." (Actually, with the mention of visions, it is worth mentioning that when students start to experiment with healing the aura and chakras they find intuition comes flooding in and that can be confusing and unsettling. Spikenard helps to steady this flow and makes it easier to comprehend.)

I have always found it easiest to think of Saturn by its name "Dweller on the threshold" because that helps me to see this is simply a long slow step but I am going into a new "house", a new space in my life. This is just settling up my account before I leave. Saturn makes you attend to every duty and responsibility before you can move on, but when you do, debts have been paid and the future looks better.

I suppose the nicest thing about Saturn is probably the same as the worst! It takes away choices. As a kid you were much more likely to do your chores and homework when you were grounded. Your best friend's party would have been far more exciting, but you just aren't allowed to go. Furious you may be, but that maths revision got done, didn't it?

Saturn, baby.

Spikenard is the antidote.

Archetype

Carl Jung first devised his system of archetypes because he noticed that his patients often described these universal stories when they had recounted their dreams to him. How could they, he wondered, all have the same meanings to each person, when these same people had never studied classical literature and had no prior knowledge of the tales at all?

These symbols are universal. They are practical, and rather than being metaphysical they are allegories for things that we all understand regardless of our creed or culture. They are inherent in all of our physiological compositions.

He noticed too, these dream often involved alchemy, again something that most people could not possibly have any firsthand knowledge about. Given that, he felt that alchemy could be an excellent tool to enable people to understand the journey of consciousness. Here, we are interested in the yellow stage of the soul's evolution, what is known as the Phoenix Stage.

Phoenix

There are two main accounts of the Phoenix.

The first is that it lived in India and that one day it flies to the frankincense tree to fill his wings with spices. Then in early spring a priest at Heliopolis covers an altar with twigs. The bird comes to the city, sees the altar, lights the fire and is entirely consumed by it. The next day a sweet worm is found in the ashes, on the second day the worm is transformed into small bird and on the third day the Phoenix has completely risen again.

In the second tale the bird lives in Arabia near a cool well. Every day, it sings the most ecstatic song. Even the sun god Apollo is so entranced by the melody that he slows his chariot to hear the bird sing. Legends differ describing his appearance. He may be red or purple, but what is sure is that there is *only ever one Phoenix in existence*. He lives for 500 years, (or maybe 540, 1000, 1461 or even 12994 years depending on whichever source you choose – regardless it is a very long time). He lives on dew and aromatic spices. He kills nothing, nor crushes nothing as he touches it. He flies around the world gathering all the wisdom he can in his existence. Then, as he senses he is aging and his end may be nigh, he builds a magnificent pyre from spikenard twigs and climbs upon it.

He turns to face the sun, his wings outstretched. Some voices tell of him starting the fire himself, banging his beak hard onto a rock igniting a spark. Others claim the heat of the sun's rays to be the catalyst. His enormous wings fan the flames until he is entirely ablaze. The bird is burned. From the ashes though, a new bird appears. When he is strong enough, the Phoenix gently lifts the nest, his father's tomb, from atop its palm tree, flies and delivers it to the temple at Heliopolis.

The archetype of the Phoenix best tells the tale of the healing given by spikenard, but strangely it has also become an allegory for Christ's resurrection from the dead. You will notice how the bird is again made flesh after three days.

The Phoenix is a powerful symbol of resurrection. He is self rejuvenating as he reincarnates. Through the baptism of the flames, its form change but its fire-like qualities remain.

Throughout humankind the bird is known, as are his qualities and he is always connected to the sun. Only his name is changed. The Chinese know the firebird as Feng Huang, the

Japanese as Ho-oo, The Russians call him Yel, and he is the Native American Thunderbird atop the totem pole. The Persians knew him as Simorg and the Indians as Semendar. To the Shamans he is Keeper of the Fires of Creation and Protector of All Fire.

In 1782 the USA gave the Phoenix a unique the Phoenix position of office upon the Great Seal. Pictured with a shield, a banner tells us *E pluribus unum* ("Out of Many, One"). It was only in 1902 that the symbol was changed to the Eagle.

Those qualities connected to the Phoenix we can also attribute to our oil: **high virtue, grace, power, prosperity, strength, peace, purity and life.**

In Feng Shui, the Phoenix has much brighter connotations but simply the reverse of the same coin. We see the positive side of the medicine. That the Phoenix always looks out in front of him, he is scanning the landscape and distant space. Summoning Phoenix energy increases our capacity for vision enabling us to collect sensory vision about our environment and the events unfolding within it. The Phoenix, the antidote to Saturn's dull landscape burns brightly, ignites intense excitement and deathless inspiration. Its heat, raising rhakta dhatu as it soars through the air, makes the destination of its flight unimportant. The Phoenix is is just happy to be there to enjoy the flight.

Note also how there is the strange correlation between the bird collecting spikenard ready for his final sacrifice for future generations, and how Christ was seemingly anointed before he made his.

What do we know of the Saturn medicine?

There will always be sacrifice. There will be an ending and then some kind of transformation to a different type of existence. Saturn makes things old and the bird senses that his life is ending.

The wheels of change have been set in motion and there can be no turning it back.

The writer of **CeCe Wynan's** song **Alabaster Box**, Dr Janice Sjostrand, presented a whole new perspective of the story that I had not thought of before.

https://www.youtube.com/watch?v=G5zIOcBiTGg

She says "You don't know the cost, of the oil in my box". We do know the financial cost, because Iscariot complained of the 300 denarii worth. So it's a different cost she speaks of; it the *emotional* cost she has spent filling that pot over the years. The humiliation and *self initiated* sacrifice she has had to summon to earn the money to buy the oil. That's her cost. But the action is bigger, isn't it? Because the song implies that this little jar was not just any old flask; this was her insurance policy. It was how she was going to survive after her looks could no longer pay the rent. But when Jesus tells her she is forgiven, she knows she has to take a gamble on believing that is true. Her unfaltering faith says, well, no then, I have no need for this insurance, and if I believe that my sins have been washed away, then this oil, polluted by the money I gave for it, has no place in my future either. This is my repentance, and my absolute sacrifice to God. I am trusting that Jesus can make things right.

So although I did not see it before, the Alabaster Box story shows us that the strongest spikenard medicine is in play again, absolute faith through sacrifice. I like this too, because it's a nice demonstration that your sacrifice will be different to mine, and I might not even recognise your sacrifice will have been made, although it will have stung *you* to the core.

In Egypt, the Phoenix is a fiery image of rebirth, again known by a different name. He is the Bennu, or known as Ben. The extraordinary Bennu had vibrant red and golden plumage, and he was the sacred bird of Heliopolis. To you and I, there might be a distinct look of a heron about him. He has an elegant and strong straight back. Adorned at the back, his majestic head is decorated by two erect feathers. Centuries later, the Greeks changed the sacred bird's name from Benn to Phoenix.

In his home of Heliopolis, the Bennu had an extremely important role to play in Egyptian mythology. His sanctuary was the ben-ben stone or obelisk within Heliopolis and he was worshipped alongside Ra and Ausar (Osiris). This City of the Sun was where the Egyptians believed the work of creation had begun. The ben-ben stood high up on the rocky mound and came to represent the first being **to arise from the primordial water chaos of creation.** His was the cry that marked the beginning of time which is why he became **ruler of time**, or minutes, days, months and years.

The image of the Bennu is the hieroglyph we have come to understand as directly representing the name of Re, the sun deity. Legend has it that the bird created itself from the fire that burned on the top of the sacred Persea tree in Heliopolisan. There is a beautiful artefact called the Metternich Stele in the Egyptian Collection of the Metropolitan Museum of Art in New York City. Hewn from stone it dates to around 350BC. It was created after a priest saw engravings at Heliopolis and wanted to copy them for means of healing. Priests would recite rituals whilst pouring water over the Stele and then would collect it for their patient to drink. The stone was ostensibly to protect the Egyptians against dangerous animals such as crocodiles and scorpions. On it, Isis says to her son, Horus *'Thou art the Great Bennu who was born on the Incense Trees in the House of the Great Prince in Heliopoli.'*

The Bennu is quintessentially linked with the sun. As it rose, 'soul of Ra,' took the form of the Bennu to shine out across the world, each morning renewed. The Bennu was thought to be Osiris made manifest and was said to "spring from his heart as a *living symbol of the god*".

The *'Book of the Dead'* is a set of 15th BCE funeral rites and therein we find formulae to transform deceased loved ones into the Great Bennu. The deceased announces, *'I am the Bennu, the soul of Ra, and the guide of the gods in the Duat.'* Later another verse tells us, *'I am pure. My purity is the purity of the Great Bennu which is in the city of Suten-henen.'*

In the 5th century BC, Herodotus recorded his thoughts about the Bennu, saying he had never seen the bird but he knew it to make its appearance only once in 500 years -- as coming from Arabia, carrying in its beak an egg of myrrh that contained its father's body. There he deposits it onto the altar of the sun god and it is consumed.

It has been suggested that the Egyptians may have caught sight of a Goliath Heron, a very rare visitor to Egypt. There has also been archaeological discoveries of remains of an even larger heron in the Gulf of Persia which is thought to be have been around 5000 years old. Another suggestion is suggested that they may have seen a flamingo from East Africa. These nest on salt flats, too hot for its eggs or chicks to survive. To protect them, the flamingo builds a mound several inches tall to support the egg in a marginally cooler location. From a distance the convection currents around the mounds look like the turbulence of a flame. (Interestingly the Linnaean classification for a flamingo is: *Phoenicopterus!*)

To the Egyptians, Bennu was the very essence of rebirth. Rising from its ashes, a new spiritual form rises to replace the the now dead physical form. As the spirit ascends it becomes the soul of Osiris made manifest.

There is something very Saturnic about the story of the Phoenix. It must have a lonely existence, for the bird truly is alone in his species, and yet he sings. For another of his kind to enter the world, he must sacrifice himself. Yet, paradoxically he is the most Saturnic medicine. In the planet's icy coldness, he is warmth, just as the spikenard is.

Alchemy

The subject of alchemy was quintessentially interested in transformation. Depending on where you lived in the world in the Middle Ages, alchemy meant different things. In Europe, alchemists became obsessed with the idea that metals could be changed. Their theory was gold had evolved through various processes in the Earth and as such, it must be possible to change lead into gold through some kind of external processing. In the East, particularly in India, alchemy was entirely plant based and in effect is the herbal medicine we use today. Their elixirs and spagyrics form the extraordinary healing still revered a millennium later. (We talk about this in detail in my Holy Basil book, you may recall).

The Rosicrucian teachings are a combination of occultism and other religious beliefs and practices, including Hermeticism, Jewish mysticism, as well as the Christian Gnosticism which surrounds the stories of the apocrypha we spoke of earlier. The central feature of Rosicrucianism was the ethos that members possessed some degree of secret wisdom handed down to them from ancient times. (Freemasonary was a later offshoot of the followers.) Rosicruicians perceived alchemy to be yet a different thing again. That, where physical alchemy (with metals and plants) was concerned with altering properties with matter, spiritual alchemy is concerned with freeing your spiritual self from being trapped within unrefined parts of your being. These parts might be fear, self loathing, doubt, and, of course, one's own personal belief about oneself and the ones own environment.

(It is provocative but interesting to state that Francis Bacon, teacher and advisor to Franklin and Washington, so by extension to the Founding Fathers, was a Rosicrucian and Freemason. I wonder then, how much of this alchemical symbology of struggle and transformation was wrapped up in that early representation of the Great Seal?)

The objective of spiritual alchemy is to achieve some kind of liberation from the core wounds that lead to day to day damage and unhappiness in one's existence. This might require some kind of transformation of a core belief system, perhaps experiencing a soul loss, and at the centre, addressing aspects of one's own destructive personality. To the Rosicrucian's the transmutation of lead into gold was nothing more than a metaphor for helping the human soul on its journey to a becoming a more perfect spirit soul. When asked about his own thoughts about the subject, Jung described how he felt alchemy must have two aims: *"To rescue the human soul and the salvation of the cosmos"*.

In spiritual alchemy, the soul passes through colour stages as it matures and changes. The Phoenix rules the yellow stage of decay and rebirth. As one would imagine, like everything connected to spikenard and the Phoenix, this can be viewed in two ways.

Yellow has the brightness of spring flowers, of the yolk of an egg, of sunlight and honey and the ripening of grains (Hello arista, our grain of animal feed!), but it is also the colour of putrification and of corruption.

The yellow stage of alchemy signals **a time for change**, usually for the worse. It is the withering of leaves, and the aging of pages, of long stored linen, of old teeth and toenails. Yellow is liver spots and peeling skin. It is the indelible stains of food and semen that no manner of detergent will shift.

The alchemist's dictum is that yellow is the sign of decay perceived by the eyes and the nose. I think that as aromatherapists we should pause for a second and notice that the olfactory distinction is important here.

This is rotting. It is ended. It is time for it to change and for something new to take its place. The motto for the yellow stage is *Solve et coagula* – break down and separate – happens in a bid to bring things back together in a higher form.

In the alchemical system, one was aspiring toward whiteness, a purity of spirit, but conversely, achieving whiteness was seen not living in completeness. It is too easy. It's clean and simple, but it lacks introspection and as such it falls short of spiritual maturity. It is only by the spilling of blood and the passing through the yellow stage that one can truly begin to live well.

This increase of white to yellow is an increase of heat (Pressure and friction always causes heat.)

Under Pressure: **David Bowie and Queen**
https://www.youtube.com/watch?v=YoDh_gHDvkk

It's through this heat we also start to have an awareness that begins to turn outward from the inside to the outside world. I suppose that it is human nature not to notice or look outward when life is easy. It is only when the heat is turned up that begin to get an awareness of what is going on outside. Its rising challenges make us sharper, more aware and often a damn site more compassionate of everyone else's challenges and choices.

And so whilst the yellowing stage of our alchemical spiritual journey might feel like a step back, it is this reflection that is required to understand exactly what work needs to be done to rectify our situation (whether that be external marital financial etc, or internal – alleviating stressors).

Before the yellow stage, or Saturn's medicine, really we suffer ignorance, and as the pain lifts we enjoy the blessing of understanding. The yellow stage, the Phoenix moment, in their Saturnic medicine bring the pain of understanding, and with it the souls suffers this understanding, but with it comes knowledge and acceptance.

And that truly is the medicine of spikenard.

I have spent many hours trying to sum up the exact vibration of spikenard. I can tell you, it is the prescribed oil for dread. It would be the best choice for someone feeling overwhelmed. Certainly it is magical against terror. But the only word I can really come up with to describe what it does..is...absence.

It brings about an absence of terror. Does that mean you become brave? No, I don't think it does. It just means you are not scared any more. In the same way, I have seen it bring about an absence of fury. One day incandescent rage, the next day, I wasn't happy, but the fury had gone. When life is overwhelming and a tidal wave of panic overcomes you, then spikenard....well, I suppose Moses might tell you it could part the Red Sea!!! I would be the last person to argue.

It dissipates.

For an oil with such a dramatic history, it is not dramatic in any way. It's calm and resolute. It reminds me of an old saying my mum uses "No fuss, no muss."

If I had to give it an emotion...and that would make it easier for matching against molecules of emotion...I would say it is the molecule of..

Let it be...

The **Beatles:** *https://www.youtube.com/watch?v=9VoRAZdc85I*

Acceptance, I suppose. No, more than that.

Spikenard brings about *acquiescence – reluctant acceptance without protest*.

Worwood says forgiveness, and certainly, that would be true. In these cynically dark days of the Twenty First century we are encouraged to rage against the machine, and to a point, certainly, fighting for your rights of freedom, liberty or at the very least respect, is the right thing to do. But at the same point at what point does it stop being healthy to be so "inflamed". When does righteous indignation become toxic not only the mind, the spirit but the physical body too?

At some point we must find a way to come to peace with what *is*. We simply have to come to terms with it. We need to do what needs to be done, but more difficultly I think, it is necessary to find a way to be OK with it, because if we let it gnaw away at us, we will be eaten up from the inside. Sooner or later, we will break, and that's too big a price to pay.

We heard Irene Cara sing about being on her own. Regardless of the small number in the cast though, life has to continue. We have jobs to do. We might as well find a way to smile though it. Spikenard helps us cope with the drudgery, his Phoenix medicine warming us in the cold and helping us to learn these arduous and painful Saturnic lessons.

The Show Must Go On - Queen

https://www.youtube.com/watch?v=5TXXbd4Tjoc

When I think of spikenard, it summons up the vibration of peacefulness in the face of adversity; something I struggle to comprehend. It makes me think of Mandela in his cell, and for that matter Terry Waite, their steadfast strength, their dignity, their silent protest. I think of the quiet, graceful power of Ghandi and the peaceful ministry of Mother Theresa.

Silent, gentle and enormously powerful.

Mahatma Ghandi once said, "The weak can never forgive. Forgiveness is the attribute of the strong." It's not an easy thing, but for the sake of our sanity, for the sake of our families, for the sake of the very cells reverberating in our bodies, we need to find a way to be that strong. I believe that spikenard can show that way.

But it is more than that, because the Phoenix has become an allegory of Christ *willingly* going to his crucifixion and we must not forget that spikenard was there on both occasions. Was its vibrartion a reminder of duty, perhaps, or birthright, or maybe even karma? And we are back to Saturn again.

There is no escaping the connection is there?

And, actually, *that* is Saturnic too. *No,* you *can't* escape the lesson you have been sent here to learn. This is *it*. *This* is your purpose. This is what every heartbeat of this existence has been preparing you for, and whether you remember all you have been taught or not, it is innate and you *will* know what to do when you get there.

For both Christ and the Phoenix, it is important to remember the saturnic promise, and spikenard is a wonderful reminder of this...*this is not the end*. There is something else waiting for you. This is merely a transition, painful as this time is, this is little more than a doorway to a different place.

Let spikenard hold your hand.

Remember though, the same divine medicine that perhaps Christ and our Phoenix experienced. And given the opening passage of this book, I can't help but think of Frodo Baggins, that tiny Hobbit who is the *only* creature capable of destroying "The Ring" too. There *is* only you who can do this. You are on your own, and that is *exactly* as it should be, because this will be your strongest moment. Potentially it is your birthright. It is what you came to do. This will be your glory.

It is most certainly one of the most divine of all the oils, (along with Holy Basil). I wonder then, whether the molecule it summons within our core might be the faith to say *"so be it"*

Perhaps its vibration is best described as *Amen*.

Leonard   *Cohen:*   *Amen:*
https://www.youtube.com/watch?v=MsYd08wQGil

God, grant me the serenity to accept the things I cannot change, Courage to change the things I can, And wisdom to know the difference.

Reinhold Niebuhr (1892–1971).

The Names of Spikenard

The word *Valeriana* can be first found in the writings of the ninth and tenth centuries. Spikenard is also known by the name *Muskroot*.

- Greek: Narden
- Latin: Nardoon
- Hindi Balchur/ Jatamansi
- Persian: Bekh –i-sanbal
- Tamil: Narti
- Bootean- Pampé (Bhutan)

The term *nard* was used by the Ancients to designate any Indian essence, rather as the term Attar is now.

Native to the Himalayan mountains, the plant grows wild in India, Nepal, Bhutan, and Sikkim, at elevations between 11,000 and 17,000 feet.

Ancient texts may have referred to it as muskroot, perhaps not only because of the the fragrance that the root has but also because it is the favourite dinner of the Siberian Musk Deer, which sadly is now a threatened species because of the precious musk it produces in a sac close to its genitals.

Moschus moschiferus has coarse grey-brown hair and lives in Siberia, China and Tibet. It grazes on spikenard and other sweet plants. The use of musk is extensive in perfumery but is also used in Chinese, Russian and Indian traditional medicines as a stimulant and antispasmodic. Historically it has also been used in treatments for spasms and to lower fever.

In 1979, a CITES order was placed on the musk pouches making it illegal to trade from them. Since then a synthetic musk has been used in perfumery. Predictably for a species such as *Homo erectus* (I won't use *sapiens* because that stipulates that these people need to *think*) there is still a large poaching industry surrounding these beautiful silent creatures.

Strange really, because to me, it looks like the properties seem mainly to come from the fodder it has been grazing upon.

Common Confusions

There are many plants on the Earth, now referred to as spikenard so just for clarity, we will review these.

American Spikenard - *Aralia Racemosa* – Found in North America, this has bitter roots and is considered by American writers to be as valuable a medicine as sasparilla is

Small spikenard - *Aralia Nudicaulis* also known as False sarsaparilla and Wild sarsaparilla. Indigenous to North

America, it is a gentle stimulant and diaphoretic. It is useful for treatments of rheumatism, syphilis, and cutaneous infections. These are the same applications as common sarsaparilla

Ploughman's spikenard - *Inula Conyza* – common names are: *Baccharis, Conzya, Conzya squarosa, Great Fleabane*

We have this one in England. It is a pretty flower that looks like small unopened dandelions. The yellow flowers blossom in August to October. Perennials, they like to grow in chalky and clay-filled soil.

The root and leaves are used in ointments and against itching and farcy (an inflammation found on animals) and in can be placed in wine to protect against jaundice.

Jamaica Spikenard- *Ballota suaveolens*

A strong scented emmenagoguic, this is also has anti hysteric, anti epileptic, expectorant and vermifuge properties. Externally it is vulnerary and an infusion of the plant can be used to treat dropsy and gravel (to us: oedema and kidney stones).

Roman texts also list **Asarum europeaum** which is translated as *wild spikenard* or *wild ginger*. leaves like a. This is a quite well known ground cover plant for shady areas in Britain having big lily pad leaves with tiny purple flowers and is more commonly recognised by the name: *asarabacca.*

The *"False Nard of Dauphine"* is still used as a charm in Switzerland. This is the root of *Anima victorialis.* The root is almost identical in appearance to true nard but has no fragrance.

Ecological Concerns

Nardostachys Jatamansi is found in natural habitats in the Himalayas from Pakistan, India, Nepal, Tibet and China. The majority, however is found in Nepal. It is a small perennial herb which grows from 10-60m in height with stout woody stocks. It grows in mountainous outcrops between 2200-4800m above sea level. In the last decade numbers of plants have declined by 75-80%.

Reconnaissance done by the **High Altitude Plant Physiology Research Centre** (HAPPRC) at Srinagar-Garthwal, assessed the areas including Dayar, Hari Ki Dun, Kumwari Pass, Pawalli, Kantha, Tungnath, The Valley of The Flowers, Bedni, Bugyal, Rudranath, Medmeshwar, and other parts of the Garwahl Himalayas for numbers of remaining plants. Their studies show only a few small pockets of Nardostachys jatamansi exist.

These pockets are steadily decreasing because of:

- An increase in human population
- Over exploitation for medicinal, religious and perfumery uses
- Extensive Clearing of forests
- Over grazing of cattle sheep and yaks

Ordinarily, one would expect to see a natural regeneration and recuperation after short periods of respite from farming and collecting but seed viability from the plants is extremely low. Its seed *production* is also very low and if you add to that the fast there has been an increase of forest fires over recent years, it becomes easier to see why the species might be struggling to sustain itself.

Consequently the plant is now a protected species.

It is classed as *endangered* in

- Aruchal Pradesh
- Sikkim
- Himachal Pradesh

And *Critically Endangered* in

- Uttarakhand

Strangely, given the rather superstar status of the plant, very little has been done to address the issue of sustainability until very recently. In 1997 the Government of India and the Peoples Republic of China approached the **Convention on International Trade in Endangered Species** of **Wild Fauna (CITES)** to ask them to devise ways of protecting this most valuable resource. Measures were put into place from 8/9/97. India has now imposed a ban on mass collection or removal of plants.

Cites Appendix II designates:

Whole and sliced roots and parts of the roots, excluding manufactured parts and derivatives such as powders, pills, extracts, tonics, tea and confectionary".

The annotation seems very severe until you realise that much of the medicine we use today actually comes from *the rhizome-* the subsoil stem , not the root.

Essential oils are classified as a natural products subset of trade (that is they are not timber) in Nepal. Export value in 2004 was recorded at RS2.5 billion, about 34.2million USD. To leave the country and to maintain the extremely lucrative value chain for the Nepalese people, the plants must be processed into a derivative. Essential oils are the perfect one.

In all, the value chain employs about 15000 people in Nepal. About 14,000 people belong to community forest groups, which totals about 1/3 of the population. These are specially designed spaces where plants are cultivated and farmed in a bid to allow the wild ones to recover and regenerate. An astounding 470,000 households in Nepal are in commercial plant harvesting. These are employed to harvest legally traded natural plant medicines.

There seems to be a very interesting relationship between the altitude of people's homes and how likely they are to be collectors. Whether that is due to the lower agricultural productivity as the mountains grow higher, or due to their ability to be able to reach some of the better, high value species, is not clearly understood.

Lower on the mountainsides, in Gorka only 2% of the households are involved. This increases with altitude.

- 25% in Uhiya and Keraunja
- 35% in Sidhabas
- Nearly everyone in Checkkampar and Samagon is involved in commercial harvesting of medicinal plants.

These legal harvests in 1995, according to Olsen et al provided and income of NPR 1000-3000 (14-42 USD) per annum per household. That is a significant contribution to a household whose grocery bill comes to between NPR 1200-8000 (USD 16.8-112).

Only about 32% use collection as their main source of livelihood with the majority collecting in their spare time. When surveyed 51% of participants revealed Nardostachys jatamansi was their preferred species of plant to collect as a means of generating income.

Rhizomes collected from pastures, community forests and are sold to local traders.

The Value Chain

60% of all processed goods are sent to India. About 40% comes to the EU. Buyers, for the most part dictate the prices, although since the advent of mobile phones, harvesters are considerably more savvy about market prices now. Collectors should be able to secure between 45-60 NPP (0.6-0.8USD) per kilo.

	Costs	Selling Price	Profit

Harvester	None	50	50
Village/ District Trader	Purchase of jatamansi	60	10
Airport Traders	Jatamansi=60 G/ment royalties=15 DDT = 6 Porter transport 6 Handling and packaging =4 Storage at the airport 7 Air transport to Nepalganj 21 Storage at the airport 4 Other expenses 6	150	21
Urban Whole salers	Expenses of transport to India including the cost of getting it across the border	200	25

It is easy to see why harvesting is so popular isn't it? The fact they have no overheads, of course, does not account for how laborious a task it is. Jatamansi grows far from human settlements and so one must travel long distances to begin collecting. It will take a person between 2-5 days to collect a full 15-20kg load.

Collection of plants is entirely dependent in snowfall. Typically most harvesting takes place between June to October. Sometimes collection can be impeded by snow arriving in early autumn or in late spring, shortening the harvest period. If snow storms do come, then collection can be shortened to just eight to ten day intervals. Everyone's favourite time to collect is during monsoon season when the ground is wet so rhizomes can be easily lifted. Often families will take the opportunity to gather plants as they move their herds from pastures in the April to August herding season.

The numbers of rhizomes harvested escalate year on year, and rising *fast* at that

- 1995   14 tons dry weight
- 1995   66 tons
- 1997   125 tons

Most collectors will make five or six trips a season to make their quota. Naturally, they will collect other herbs as they go. They will sell their 90-120kg of jatamansi for NPR 5k-75k (70-104 USD)

The Cites restrictions means that supply does not even come close to the demand for jatamansi. Nardostachys grandiflora is particularly sensitive to harvest, and collectors rarely leave enough of the rhizome intact for the plant to re-establish itself. Volatiles are at their optimum levels just after the reproductive phase and since offspring set themselves so close to mature rhizomes, harvesting means young plants often get damaged too. There are supposed to be long cycles between rotations for collection, but this is very hard to regulate particularly in the higher altitude areas, where the best specimens grow, because populations of plants grow in such far flung places. Policing is difficult and illegal trading is rife.

By contrast the main areas for collection in India are Uttaranchal and Himachal Pradesh, in particular these are moist, steep and rocky habitats of 3000m above sea level or higher. Harvest takes place during April and May.

Progress to see the species beginning to re-stablish is slow. The plants naturally release seed to pollinate between 7-11am in July and August. Some drop to the floor, some are carried by the wind and insects, but still the plants cannot make enough seeds to survive. This is also affected by the fact that there are hundreds of populations all with vastly diverse genetic strains. This mainly seems to be due to environmental factors (in the soil etc) rather than because of differences altitude, nevertheless, it means that each population has to be addressed as a separate strain.

Efforts are being employed in situ and ex situ, in laboratories etc. In situ measures such as employing vigilance as to who is picking what and when, applying restrictions and of course basic measures such as putting up fences and boundaries to keep both two legged and four legged visitors out. Creation of biosphere reserves, gene sanctuaries and national parks such as The Valley of The flowers all contribute to spaces where the plant can relax, breathe and perpetuate its lifecycle and regenerate. These measures, however, can only go so far.

There are problems with relying on preservation in situ when areas are prone to seismic or volcanic activity or even soil erosion. One natural disaster and the entire species could be wiped out. Ex situ measures, then, have to be employed.

Since the reproduction of the plant is erratic, slow and unreliable there is a great deal of focus on understanding how best to process and store the seeds. It is now understood that seeds from the genus retain viability for twice the length of time if they are kept in refrigerated conditions, but then of course that requires a great deal of space allocation to be employed. Studies demonstrate that seeds should be sown in a mix of sand, soil and farmyard mature in equal parts but with twice the amount of sand when plants are planted out in October and Febuary in the middle altitudes of 1800 m, and also when they plant at higher altitudes (3800m) in May. What is interesting is that despite all these different chemotypes, the percentage of seeds that will germinate seems to be fairly consistent over each population.

Just as humans have obstacles to fertility which can be treated in vitro, experimentation is underway to overcome difficulties such as abortive embryos, low seed viability and specific germination requirements. Attempts have been made too, to make shoots grow from roots, and of course division of rhizomes.

Essential Oil Production

The collected rhizomes are then cleaned and air dried. Its quality will be affected by multiple factors:

- Growing conditions and altitude
- Maturity of the rhizomes
- Their preparation
- How well they are stored
- How long they are stored

It will take 80kg of raw material to make 1kg of oil

(Just for interest and as an approximation= if we say 1kg is the same as a litre, that means 8kg for 100 mil. 1ml = 800g = 4g of root to make that simple drop of oil to go in your bath. I would have been happy with that but The Genius Son pointed out the general consensus is 1kg weight is 1041ml by volume, so 1 drop of oil is 3.84 grams of raw product.)

In 2004 a total of 204,648kg of jatamansi was harvested. Local and national distillers consumed 153,859kg. The rest was exported to India through informal channels.

Our precious volatile oils are mostly found in the delicate fibrous hairs of the rhizome. If these are damaged then the delicate volatiles are lost.

 The best oil is thought to be obtained from rhizomes between 2-3 years old and that have been dried in the shade rather than in the sun.

Oil yields vary greatly from 0.57 -1.67 % of dry weight but it is possible to gain as much as 2.9% with a very slow distillation of 15 hours.

Part 4 Spikenard in Aromatherapy

Extraction

The essential oil is extracted by steam distillation from crushed rhizomes and roots and will yield between 1-3%.

Eden Botanicals also do a CO2 which is even deeper and earthier.

Note

Base and base to middle

Fragrance

Steffen Archtander describes the fragrance as:

Heavy, sweet woods, spicy animals, reminiscent of valerian, ginger, cardamom, Atlas cedar, with a warm spicy wood, sweetness with a pinewood bitter burning flavour. Powerful. Useful in oriental perfumery types.

I think it smells of damp rotting wood. It is dank like the forest floor it came from.

Blends well with

Mandarin, Petitgrain, Roman Camomile, Green Mandarin, Tea Tree, Lavender, Clary sage, Neroli, Vetiver, Lemon, Cedarwood, sandalwood.

Safety Data:

Generally regarded as safe. No adverse reactions reported in Tisserand and Young 2013. However, in 2012, a study was undertaken into the effects of NJ on DNA, given the widespread erroneous belief that "if it is natural it cannot hurt you."

It was found that it was genotoxic when used as an aqueous extract at 5 mg/ml and at 10 mg/ml as a hydroalcoholic extract. These are not essential oils and the jury is still out as to whether an essential oil can alter DNA so this may or may not be valuable data. I think it would be fair to say don't use it for too long without rotating it with another oil to give the body a fighting chance. The question is how long? Its out of my area of knowledge to say, but for my own part, I am going to use for up to two weeks and then take a break.

3% dilution seems to be correct, but when you read the Parkinson's clinical evidence you might decide you want to try 4-5% in severe cases.

Uses and Applications
Sedative and Anxiolytic

Of all the qualities of spikenard its sedative nature must be king. Kurt Schnaubelt rates it as the most powerful in aromatherapy. (I am not sure...I think yarrow might hold the crown, but if it does spikenard is definitely close on its tail).

In their 2009 paper Kathi Keville and Mindy Green explained how they had found that spikenard increases the growth of nerve endings called ganglions without depressing the parasympathetic nervous system. In other words, spikenard is treating the patient through a sedative action but the mind and body remain alert. Schnaubelt recommends rubbing spikenard over the heart or the solar plexus chakra to gain the most sedative effect.

Jatamansi is wonderfully calming and grounding. More importantly for regaining health after trauma, it helps you drift off and sustain deep and peaceful slumber. In that gentle state the mind relaxes into dream state, working through and releasing subconscious trauma.

Skin

Dietrich Gumbel was a pioneer in anthroposophical medicine, a strain of holistic thinking that looks as diagnosis of illnesses with a spiritual context. (Like I do really, I suppose). *Anthropos* = human being : *Sophia* = wisdom

He was eager to create a skin care range that was able to address the emotional and spiritual dimensions of dis-ease. He chose spikenard to head up the range declaring it able to rectify virtually every type of problem. He explains that spikenard is the only essential oil to find the inner balance in the emotional, spiritual and physical interplay of energies. We see that in the chakra medicine later too. It acts like a universal panacea.

Jeanne Rose agrees, regaling its hormonal, relaxing and *balancing effects on every system of organs*, including the skin. She explains how the oil redresses the skin's physiological balance and causes permanent regeneration. She feels it is of particular use for mature skin.

I have found it very useful for alleviating the torturous itching of eczema and it seems to reduce the redness and flaking of psoriasis.

Uses:

- Allergies
- Anxiety
- Back Pain
- Candida (anti fungal)

- Dandruff (Schaubelt asserts it the only oil to be able to treat this condition effectively)
- Flatulence
- Aches and Pains
- Nervous Indigestion
- Psoriasis
- Rashes
- Scars (*Although my choices would be helichrysm and jasmine)
- Sclerderma
- Haemorrhoids
- Menstrual Difficulties – smoothes flow and reduces pain
- Migraines
- Nausea
- Staphyllococcus Infections
- Stretch marks
- Tachycardia
- Tension
- Hysteria
- Varicose veins (*I'd opt for geranium in preference)
- Spiritual anxiety and loss of faith

Emotional

We have seen how the oil can help you to reach a point of forgiveness and likewise to take you to a place of inner calm. It reduces fearfulness and helps to gain perspective and equilibrium.

Kathy Padecky speaks of how it intensifies feelings of spiritual love and devotion. She recommends using it in sessions of mediation because its dissipated anger and grief.

There is certainly a sense of serenity and earthly humility to the oil, and it conveys power of devotion to one's path. (I have found that to be any path too. This sense of willpower could be revision, dieting, caring...)

Most important though must be its effects on fear and anxiety and so I wanted to investigate that mechanism in more depth. Many of you will remember a blog post I wrote a year ago, when I encountered what I can genuinely describe as the most frightening day of my life. I came home terrified to the core and almost accidentally discovered a long forgotten bottle of spikenard in the bathroom cupboard. It was that experience that made me want to study spikenard.

If you want to read it, you can find it at: http://thesecrethealer.com/2015/03/spikenard-liquid-aneasthetic/

I believe those drops of oil saved my sanity that day. Thanks to spikenard and to members of my family and friends, I remained me. But it might very easily have been a very different story, because fear has the capability to ruin lives.

I find it bizarre, that as humans, we understand electricity and atomic science better than we comprehend thoughts. No-one has ever touched or seen thoughts and yet everyone has had an idea (some better than others!) and so would not refute their existence. What they are though, how they work, remains a mystery.

Fear affects thoughts in a radical way. It plays tricks on the mind. It can misperceive threats as far higher than they are, but conversely if we have made decisions when we are frightened we might also give the threat less credence than it deserves too. Given the fact that our bodies negatively react to chronic levels stress, it might be the actual act of fretting might turn out to be far more dangerous than the threat we worry might be waiting outside of our door.

If we think back to our poor old rats over the years we can pull back some horrifying evidence. Fear and stress responses in the rodents have been associated with weakened immune system, increased cardiovascular injury, gastro-intestinal damage, ulcers, irritable bowel syndrome, decreased fertility, impaired formation of long term memories, damage to certain parts of the brain such as the hippocampus, fatigue, increased risk of osteoporosis, Type II diabetes, aggravated depression and even premature death. Now *that* is terrifying to me and that's just the physical body! The clinical trials later are proof that spikenard helps every single aspect of that list.

Fear leads to immense emotional turmoil. There may have been a memory of having been hurt leaving a dread of hurt again. It can be frightening to live and even more terrifying to imagine death. Often there can be a panic of not understanding who one is, or worse the lingering dread of discovering who we are or what we may have once been. Many of us, I am sure can recognise the dark feeling at the pit of our stomach and the fear of uncertainty of what will come to pass lurking just outside of the door.

Challenges seem bigger, overwhelming somehow. A fear I remember well from my days in an abusive relationship was a fear of not knowing the answers or perhaps not understanding the question that was going to be thrown at me each evening. There is the terror of being controlled, of freedom being taken away from us. We might be scared of what others may do to us, or have done to us in the past and will continue to do. Worse, that they might move their rage onto someone weaker and more vulnerable and suddenly fear becomes a panicked need to protect. When I eventually left that relationship, PTSD took hold and my doctors very cleverly got me into CBT and onto an awareness course for professionals about domestic violence. A story was told of a 999 call made by a neighbour to the police and ambulance service because the lady next door seemed to have suffered some kind of breakdown.

The lady was 65 and had been married to her husband for nearly 40 years. Every day he had gone through the same ritual to ensure that she had cleaned the house thoroughly. He hid 15 coins which she must present to him as she served up his dinner. For 40 years she had managed to offer them up. On this day, though, she could only find 14. The poor woman was beside herself, terrified that she would be beaten. When the husband returned home, the police discovered he had maliciously hidden one in his pocket. It transpired that no punches had ever been pulled, nevertheless the poor woman had spent the whole of her life ruled by fear. What difference would spikenard have made to *her* existence, I wonder?

Many other so called "mental disorders" also often rear their ugly heads because of a perception if fear. This fear can take many forms: of individuals or of society as a whole (in the form of the paranoia of schizophrenia for example.) In a schizophrenic state, there are *few* feelings in the body apart from fear.

As fear morphs into insidious paranoia some may become afraid of other people but worse feel they may not even *be* people. Most terrifying must be that aching concern that you are not the person others see you as, or the menacing suspicion that *you* are not a person at all.

Not all times of fear, are frightening times either. For example, in a therapy situation, we ourselves may feel anxious or fearful of not knowing what questions to ask. There will be times in our lives when we all step with trepidation.

Traumatic events can often be a catalyst and whilst many people might overcome traumatic experiences pretty much unscathed, about 20% will experience mild anxiety problems and more will suffer long term mental health problems. Having an essential oil at our disposal capable of alleviating fear is a powerful weapon to have in our arsenal.

Think of processes it can halt. Visualise how fear makes us distrustful and as we distrust, so we become even more fearful. Spikenard moves fear from the equation making intimacy easier on every level whether that might be patient and carer, parent and child, and of course a more secure union between lovers.

Challenges we might have previously taken in our stride seem insurmountable when we are afraid. Spikenard says *Stop! Think. You've done this before. You can do it again.* It helps us to feel more in control, and when we have that sense of mastery, impotence leaves us and we feel more capable of moving forward. We can quietly review our choices and that is very important to managing fear. A calculated risk we make from our own volition is far less intimidating than one imposed on us by others. (I suppose this idea of choosing do it yourself makes it a sacrifice to really, doesn't it?) Empowerment deems fear as surplus to requirement. What was is Susan Jeffers said? *"Feel the Fear and Do It Anyway"*

There is a difference too, isn't there between fear and anxiety? On the surface one seems greater than the other, but whilst fear might be of some imminent, *immediate* threat, anxiety is a lingering, chronic worry that something bad might be about to happen, even if you can't quite put your finger on what that *something* might be.

How we react to a traumatic situation is, of course, an entirely individual response. Even, I suspect are our fear associations. Just as in The Essential Oils of The Mind Body Spirit we discuss qualia and how we uniquely experience a quality or property, (such as the smell of coriander or seeing the colour green), I cannot be sure that that sinking feeling in my stomach is the same as you feel yours. What I can know is I recognise my unique cocktail of neurotransmitters as..."Something is very wrong" because I have felt it many times before.

You may or not know that one of my ghost writing jobs is to write training manuals for bank staff about how to react in armed robbery situations. You will be glad to know it is the advice of a trained police negotiator that goes onto the paper (I am pretty much paid to write the blagger's swearing and to add the science of fear). So, my thoughts regularly wander to the plight of the teller who is held up at gun point, and how they will recover day to day.

The fight or flight response is covered in detail in the Professional Stress Solution and I would urge you to re-read it. Most pertinent here is to recall that the automatic response is far faster than any conscious thought you might have. In other words, your reaction in these situations can only depend on previous learned behaviours, whether that be from a robbery training package, your life thus far, or hopefully not the fact that a relative was killed in a robbery. The ability to stay calm and collected means fear cannot overwhelm you.

There are no right or wrong ways to deal with the aftermath of trauma. Some people might suffer feelings of helplessness of not wanting to believe that it has happened, both of which are entirely understandable. These feelings may escalate, however, to extreme anxiety, fear and even despair. Some may relive the experience the trauma in the form of flashbacks, have trouble concentrating, experience extreme fear and, of course, notice an increase in health problems.

For most, anxiety will provoke several times in the oncoming months. This may trigger different emotions of guilt, shame, or even depression. If they are strong reactions, they might even feel ridiculous, as if it were out of kilter with what the person perceives a rational response might be. In most cases the effects will decrease day by day and intensity will fade away.

Long term fear, though, can be dangerous. A fear may arise many years after the trauma that caused it. A childhood trauma, perhaps. The problem being, the coping mechanism that the child used all those years ago will be the same one that surfaces now. Often it will not serve an adult well. This regression means the adult survivor adopts the role of fighter, accommodator, escape artist, victim, over-achiever, or 'pleaser'. In some cases, where the youngster has sought to repress the experience in a bid to prevent feelings overwhelming them, they may learn to disassociate. Dividing the overwhelming experiences into manageable parts helps them to feel more in command of the situation. They will reject intimacy or authority as a means of not having to trust. Clearly whilst these strategies help the person to avoid the full impact of the trauma, and thus edge away from the sensation of being helpless it becomes almost impossible for the person to live a happy, calm and integrated life.

In contrast, the child who has had a nurturing and fearless childhood will learn wholly different strategies and may be able to get though these events simply by talking them through with family and friends. Funnily enough, my own coping strategy was to put some oil in the bath which was exactly what my mum would have done for me when I was a child. Only then I would have laughed at her!

Chakra Medicine

Spikenard balances and radiates the energy of *every* chakra.

Base Chakra – As with all root oils, spikenard helps to ground a person. Especially useful if they are struggling with fear.

Sacral Chakra – This is the chakra of boundaries, very useful to work with when Saturn is teaching you to test your boundaries! Likewise though, predictably we are heading in to tantric realms of trust and intimacy.

When the sacral energy is balanced we are patient. Out of balance we are likely to see the negative side of Capricorn, suspicion, jealousy and paranoia.

Solar Plexus – useful if the person is struggling with issues with self identity. I used the example of a woman whose husband is in jail earlier. We might think of the way this oppression might make her think she appears to other people because of her situation. Clearly too, this is the chakra most connected with transformation and the colour yellow (like the alchemic stage of the Phoenix)

Don't forget too, this is the centre of will-power and discipline, just as if we were deliberately summoning Saturn's energy.

When solar plexus energy is too powerful we react to life circumstances, we have emotional outbursts. In contrast, blocked or deficient solar plexus energy makes us passive and inactive. We allow life to pass by without engaging. Spikenard tonifies the third chakra allowing us the ability to make conscious choices to choose and to act.

Heart Chakra: probably the chakra where is sits in most comfort, allowing the heart to open with empathy and compassion. This is the seat of forgiveness. Physically, and importantly, this is also the healing aspect of cardiac and respiratory wellness.

Throat Chakra: Again very useful when the situation demands you keep your opinions firmly to yourself. Helps you to find a vibration where inexpression sits better with you thus protecting you from coughs and throat issues. A powerful ally for people who cannot keep their gob shut. (Note to self: You might want to carry a few bottles with you, Elizabeth Ashley!!!)

Brow Chakra – We use it here when we want to summon an ability to see the bigger picture. Gaining insights and feeling more certain of the future. Physically, of course, we see neurological issues so one must wonder at the effects on the Parkinson's and epilepsy for example.

Crown Chakra – Connection with the divine. Pure faith. Experience without prejudice. Feeling a connectedness with the world around you, both on a physical and cosmic level.

Spikenard's influence on the crown chakra is the perfect antidote to Saturn's message that you are all alone.

Part 5 Chemistry

I am approaching this section a little differently because I want to convey the deep interconnectedness between this now-rare plant and its place in our universe. Spiritually, history has shown its divine relationship connecting Heaven and Earth. In this section, I wanted to investigate the relationship that the Nardostachys grandiflora enjoyed in its Himalayan paradise and how the way it interacts with its surroundings also impacts on our lives.

Often I will read statements like "sesquiterpenes will pass the blood brain barrier" and they fill me with trepidation. That's not enough for me. I want to understand *how*. This study seemed to be the perfect opportunity to understand the neurological healing of essential oils at a deeper level

I was interested to see not only scientific evidence in a petri dish but to also put that into a context where we can comprehend how and why plants can help alter emotional and neurological states. To that end then, I speak of plant metabolites as a whole, in line with current research, then look at specific chemical trials.

Plant Metabolites and their role in neuropharmacology

The 21st century seems riddled with concern over cognitive dysfunction. When I was speaking for the IFA in Beijing last year, I heard Dr Marilyn Glenville speak about how Alzheimer's Syndrome may be renamed Type III diabetes because the fat receptors in our bellies actually work as organs independently attacking the brain. That was enough to put me on a diet!

Neuropsychiatric disorders and neurodegenerative disorders, such as schizophrenia, depression, Alzheimer's Disease dementia, cerebrovascular impairment, seizure disorders, head injury and Parkinsonism are so debilitating in nature, I think I would do anything to avoid their horrible visitations. Research into this area fascinates me, not least because the research seems so closely related to psychoneuroenocrinology and our Mind-Body Spirit medicine. Over the past decade, many neurotransmitters and signalling molecules have been identified as possible therapeutic targets. Some are conventional or synthetic molecules, but since between a quarter to a half of medicines have plant derived sources, many are phytochemicals extracted from medicinal plants. These play a vital role in maintaining chemical balance in the brain by influencing the function of receptors and then attaching to the major inhibitory neurotransmitters.

Clearly, our brains are the the most complex structure in our bodies. They are comprised of *neurons* and *neuroglia* (these are neurons whose job is to send and receive nerve impulses and signals.)

In addition the proper functioning of the neurons is overseen by the fast acting responses of microglia (macrophage cells that hunt out, warrior-like, any infection in the brain) and *astrocytes*. Astrocytes are neuroglials, (or glial cells) whose function is to bring the body into homeostasis. They form the protective sheath surrounding our nerves called myelin. Although their names are unfamiliar to most of us, they are ultimately responsible for brain (and by extension holistic) health. Their damage or impairment has devastating consequences for brain function.

Our understanding of the brain is still very limited but it is thought that neuroglial activation is largely determined by this neuronal signalling. Any acute injury will trigger neurons to generate signals informing neuroglia of the impaired neuronal status. Depending on how bad the neuronal injury is, neuroglia might choose to either nurse the injured neurons into better health or slaughter them because they are no longer viable. These responses represent normal physiological and neuroprotective responses.

By contrast, some chronic processes perpetually activate these neuroglia eventually damaging their capacity to maintain homeostasis.

Neuro-degeneration happens in neuropathological conditions but it will also happen naturally as the brain ages and cerebrovascular and neurogenerative dysfunction accounts of 8% of total death rate in our species. Finding neuroprotective strategies able to defend the central nervous system against neuronal injury due to both acute (e.g. stroke or trauma) and chronic neurodegenerative disorders (e.g. Alzheimer's disease and Parkinson's disease) will greatly enhance the quality of human life.

You will see as we enter the clinical research section, just how great a degree the health authorities are motivated by this. Our plant medicine stands at the very centre of their efforts.

Medical drugs and nutritional supplements exerting positive effects on brain function fall under the branch of pharmacology called *Nootropics*; (pronounced *no-oh-trohpic*).

The word comes from Greek νόος (nóos, "mind") and τροπέω and means "acting on the mind." These drugs generally work by altering the balance in the levels of neurotransmitters active in the brain. The beauty of medicinal plants is rather than having side effects they have many main effects. Containing literally millions of metabolites and secondary metabolites, these are able to target many actions at a time. Whilst being wonderful, this also means understanding how a plant fully provides its medicine becomes ever more complex.

Psychoactive properties of these medicines derive from presence of plant secondary metabolites. These are chemicals unrequired for the immediate survival of the plant but they are synthesized in order to increase the fitness of the plant. They ensure its survival by allowing it to interact with its environment repelling pathogens and insects that might gobble them up and attracting pretty butterfly feet and bumbling bees. One interesting question we might want to ask ourselves is how is it that a plant can have metabolites that affect human brain function? After all the species are entirely different.

There are two possible answers. The first is that plants and animals may be less different than they seem. The second may be that organically we may be quite similar to the insects who interact with the plants, and thus we react in a similar way.

Nootropics affect the mind by acting in a variety of ways, some by enhancing cerebral blood flow, others influence the rate the brain metabolises oxygen and cerebral glucose, others still work by aiding the memory through a large number of different channels.

Apart from the obvious advantages of a healthier medicinal way, cynically we must also consider the fiscal benefits of creating plant medicines for drug companies. The general population now conceives naturally derived substances and extracts as being safer and more desirable than synthetic chemical products, which means herbal preparations are also guaranteed to have cash registers ringing. Paradoxically though, whilst herbal extracts are literally rushing off the shelves, they are supported by a dearth of scientific evidence, whilst the drug companies are still concentrating on synthetic options. It might appear from books like mine that there many clinical trials, but whilst they are undoubtedly growing, the numbers are still tragically few in the West. India, with Nardostachys in particular, is leading the way.

There are more than 120 traditional medicines being used for the therapy of CNS disorders in Asian countries. Ayurvedic neuropsychopharmacology research shows potential for *Allium sativum, Bacopa monnierae, Centella asiatica, Celastrus paniculatus, Nicotiana tabaccum, Withania somnifera, Ricinus communis, Salvia officinalis, Ginkgo biloba, Huperiza serrata, Angelica sinensis, Uncaria tomentosa, Hypericum perforatum, Physostigma venosum, Acorus calmus, Curcuma longa, Terminalia chebula, Crocus sativus, Enhydra fluctuans, Valeriana wallichii,*

Glycyrrhiza glabra, to name but a few, as well as our *Nardostachys jatamansi* of course.

Likewise in Chinese medicine, numerous plants are being researched to assess the validity of their traditional reputations of treating strokes, for example: *Ledebouriella divaricata, Scutellaria baicalensis, Angelica pubescens, Morus alba, Salvia miltiorrhiza, Uncaria rhynchophylla, and Ligusticum chuanxiong.*

Much of the research into plants relies on their anti-oxidant effects. Oxidative stress, injuring neuronal cells, is implicated in many mechanisms of pathological states of the brain, which would also include neurodegenerative disorders.

Although the brain accounts for less than 2% of the body weight, its functions burn about 20% of the oxygen made available from respiration. Given this then, the brain is extremely vulnerable to oxidation, but has a very limited capability to counteract this oxidative stress. Its high oxygen demand means the brain is the more susceptible to oxidative damage than any other organ in the body.

Central nervous system cells can fight oxidative stress if they herald resources available from food sources such as vitamins and antioxidant enzymes, but this defence system can be activated/ improved by nutritional antioxidants such as polyphenols, flavonids, terpenoids, fatty acids etc.

Anti-oxidants work by scavenging free radicals. They act by donating an electron to cells, thus making them more stable. Plant derived *alternative antioxidants* (you will see this written as AOX) are seen as effective in controlling the effects of oxidative damage. This influences what people eat and drink these days, a great deal. The smoothies we see in Starbucks for ridonculous amounts of pennies for instance, are recognised by the general public as being beneficial to health.

Empirical evidence supporting the use of antioxidants for the control of neurodegenerative disorders is vast now and again we see its influence in spikenard research, not least because the focus of medicine is shifting from treatment to prevention of disease as a means not only to elongate life, but also remove pressure from the overburdened health services.

It seems most likely that plants become neuro-protective and neuro-regenerative by protecting against this oxidation of cells; by reducing or reversing cell damage and thereby slowing progression of neuronal cell loss although their action is still not fully understood and we wait patiently for further elucidation.

A variety of plant derived flavonoids, terpenes, and related substances affect the function of ionotropic GABA receptors. (for example grapefruit and are known to cross that blood brain barrier

Here are some of the main active components found in essential oils and other plant derivative acting on the central nervous system in therapy.

Phenols

In the 1990s there was a sudden surge in interest in phenolic compounds in foods. Evidence from studies and clinical trials had shown that polyphenols from apple, grape, and citrus fruit juices possessed stronger neuroprotective properties than antioxidant vitamins. In the clinical research, you will see that Nardostachys Jatamansi offers profound antioxidant properties and this is due, for the most part to its phenolic content.

Phenols are involved in repelling creatures from eating them, but for the most part they have a gentler part to play in the co-existence with the cosmos. Phenols will be triggered in a plant if it faced with bacterial or fungal attack, for example. They defend the plant. They provide it with its rich scents, vibrant colors, and flavours to seduce symbiotic insects, but to also deter herbivores. Phenolic compounds manage soil bacteria.

Alongside these roles, many of these compounds also play roles in antioxidant defences as well as managing the absorption of UV light.

In terms of central nervous system function, a wide range of phenolic compounds interact directly with neurotransmitter systems. Many rodent studies models have demonstrated that berry extracts with high levels of anthocyanins or other polyphenols have the capability to reverse brain injuries and-and age-related cognitive decline. More pertinently to us, these studies proved that polyphenols are able to cross the blood brain barrier. This mechanism is potentially the most important aspect of why plant medicine may become so important. The barrier protects against foreign objects (xenobiotics) by making it almost impossible to cross. Imagine it like a very tightly knitted mesh. To pass through it molecules must be incredibly small. Many chemotherapies for instance are useless on the brain, since their molecules are too large to penetrate the BBB.

Polyphenols identified in a 2015 study by the Defence Food Research Laboratory in Mysore included:
Gallic acid (0.18 mg/g), catechin (4.37 mg/g), chlorogenic acid (19.90 mg/g), homovanillic acid (32.02 mg/g), epicatechin

(4.23 mg/g), rutin hydrate (0.08 mg/g) and quercetin-3-rhamnoside (7.13 mg/g).

They added that they felt other phenols were also present but because of a lack of comparative data they had been unable to identify them.

More recently interest has also grown into what the potential might be in modulating neuronal function and prevent age-related neurodegeneration through the medium of flavonoids. Where there have been animal studies into supplementation of diet with these secondary plant metabolites they have been found to protect vulnerable neurons, enhance existing neuronal function and to stimulate neuronal regeneration thus improving memory and learning.

In order for flavonoids to access the brain, again they must first cross the blood brain barrier (BBB), and flavanones such as hesperetin, naringenin and their *in vivo* metabolites have been shown to cross the BBB in relevant *in vitro* and *in situ* models.

Similarly, there is evidence of mixtures of cocoa-flavanols increasing peripheral vaso-dilation and cerebral blow flow during concentration when it has been scanned with an MRI. Further the cocoa showed improved performance on cognitively demanding tasks, so it has been suggested that flavonoid-rich foods may limit neurodegeneration and prevent or reverse normal or abnormal deteriorations in cognitive performance.

Animal studies show individual and combined flavonoids found in traditional medicinal extracts exert sedative/anxiolytic effects by direct binding to $GABA_A$ receptors. Cognitive processing is enhanced via antagonistic $GABA_A$ receptor binding and resultant cholinergic upregulation. One of the mechanisms suggested to affect dementia is decreased cholinergic activity in brain. You will meet this is more depth in a moment. This is a growth area of research because many plant derived cholinergic drugs are already in general circulation as a means of improving memory. Antidepressant effects are achieved by via monoamine oxidase inhibition which results in increases in levels of 5-HT, dopamine, and noradrenaline in various areas of the brain. Phytochemicals modify neuronal excitability either by activating or inhibiting specific receptors or ion channels.

Flavonones have also been found to have MAO inhibitory activity, which again we will investigate in a moment.

Alkaloids are a huge chemical group of containing carbon, nitrogen, hydrogen and usually a bit of oxygen. They are found in over 20% of plant species. Although no single classification exists, alkaloids are often distinguished on the basis of a structural similarity (e.g. indole alkaloids) or a common precursor (e.g. benzylisoquinoline, tropane, pyrrolizidine, or purine alkaloids).

We can trace the recorded use of alkaloids for medicinal purposes back some 5000 years because this is chemical group has contributed most of the poisons, neurotoxins, and traditional psychedelics of recorded history (e.g. atropine, scopolamine, and hyoscyamine, from the plant *Atropa Belladonna*) as well as social drugs like nicotine, caffeine, methamphetamine (ephedrine), cocaine, and opiates so desirous to humans .

The ecological role of an alkaloid is to primarily act as a feeding deterrent or toxin to any insects or other munching creature. Usually this chemical component will interact directly with molecular targets in the nervous system. Individual alkaloids act as agonists and antagonists to a variety of neurotransmitter systems by binding to neuroreceptors and interfering with neurotransmitter metabolism (e.g. this is what we will see with cholinesterase inhibition). Sometimes effects can be through signal transduction or ion channel function or it might mimic the structure of endogenous neurochemicals already in the system

It's interesting to visualise what these alkaloids will do to the plant's predator (You can tell I have got a six year old boy...my imagined herbivore is a stagasaurus! Only about 150 million years out, Liz! For jatamansi, try a yak! Anyway...)

The nature of plant-derived alkaloids is to be toxic to mammals (although there are some specialized herbivorous species which have evolved and adapted to tolerate them.) Hagen et al. hypothesized that the psychoactive effects of alkaloid addictive drugs may be derived from their ecological role as insect deterrents and as such toxins, and suggests that their addictive properties may partly arise as a consequence of the divergence of some of the roles of dopamine in insects and mammals as the relative species have evolved.

Research shows that alkaloids affect the CNS through nerve cells of the brain and through the spinal cord thus affecting physiology and behaviour. It is possible they may also affect the autonomic nervous system, thus regulating internal organs, heartbeat, circulation and breathing. These alkaloids may interfere or compete with the action of serotonin in the brain.

Ergot alkaloids have marked effects on blood flow, which was originally thought to be the main mechanism of their action. *Tropane alkaloids* like *atropine*, our deadly nightshade friend *scopolamine* (usually used in memory trials) and the spinal cord. The most famous *iso-quinoline alkaloid* must surely be morphine, (isolated from *Papaver somniferum* or the opium poppy) used as aa potent analgesic and,, of course a narcotic drug. Galantamine is a tertiary alkaloid, belonging to the phenanthrene chemical class, which occurs naturally in the daffodil (*Narcissus tazetta*), snowdrop (*Galanthus nivalis*) and the snowflake (*Leucojum aestivum*). The drug also belongs to a class of drugs called cholinesterase inhibitors and is capable of stimulating nicotinic receptors which further enhance cognition and memory. Again, you will meet this in the next part.

Terpenoids

Terpenes are a diverse group of more than 30,000 lipid-soluble compounds. From a caterpillar point of view these are somewhat unpredictable exhibiting a range of toxicity from deadly to entirely edible. They have a broad range of ecological roles, including antimicrobial properties and a massive toolbox of lovelies to that attract allies for to pollinate and spread seed for them. These enable the plant to emit airborne chemical signals and scents, flavour, and taste. Monoterpenes can also function as antigerminative or phytotoxic agents as well as influencing growth. Since the terpenes also exhibit a wide range of effects upon the predatory insect CNS. It could be of course that the metabolites work on our systems because are evolutionarily similar to them! For instance, the neurotoxic deterrent properties of many monoterpenes in insects have been shown to interact with their GABA receptors, the same way as it does on ours. Plants also synthesize a wide range of insect hormones and thus may play a defensive role by interfering with the life course and reproductive behaviour of the muchers. Metabolites will, for instance, affect the regularity of pupation, metamorphoses, and molting in some caterpillars.

Meanwhile other phytochemicals will act as either deterrent or attractant. One of these you will recognise is 1,8-cineole, the "problematic" component in eucalyptus which makes it difficult to use on children, but that actually does all the medicinal magic. It is also found in sage and melissa extracts. It acts as a toxin to beetles and some species of flies but it is harmless to some other honeybees acting as a fragrant seduction to honey bees for insect pollination. It is interesting to note that many terpenoids, very toxic to some insects, have very low toxicity for mammals. In this particular sector we find spices, flavours, and foods that form essential components of our diets both in terms of the provision of taste and healthy eating. Relevantly too, monoterpenes tend to work the most synergistically with other components in the plant supporting one another and add to the total strength of the plant. Three terpenoid compounds isolated which are nardal, jatamansic acid, nardin and Nardostachysin.

Th largest group of constituents you will find in Nardostachys grandiflora is sesquiterpenes. *Jatamansone* and *valeranone* are the principal sesquiterpene.

(The other sesquiterpenes include: Alpha-patcho-ulense, angelicin, β-eudesemo, β- atchoulense, β-sitosterol, calarene, elemol, jatamansin, jatamansinol [15], jatamansone, n-hexaco-sanyl, n-hexacosane, Oroselol, patchouli alcohol, valeranal, valeranone, nardostachnol, seychellene, seychelane, nardostachone.)

Until 1966, essential oils containing mono- and sesquiterpinoids were believed to only have a sedative effect. Because of the Valerinacea genus, the entire face of pharmacology was about to change. Schültz and Müller and Mannetstätter were the first to isolate a new group of active compounds. Latterly, this group was then characterised by Thies et al. Theis gave these the name of **Valepotriates** derived from *Valeriana epoxytriester*.

Initial trials revealed that somewhere between sedation and tranquilisation there existed a new, never before seen, action. The term "*aequilans*" describes this activity meaning that valpotriates are less useful as sleep inducing drugs, but more so as sedatives. They have a specific dampening effect on the central nervous system which works together with improving motor co-ordination. In 1981 these valepotriates were also identified as having extreme cytotoxic potential.

Indian Valerian (*wallichii*) contains four times as many valepotriates than the European equivalent (*officinalis*) (2% in comparison to 0.5%) but the component "valeranone" is also found in jatamansi. In animal studies its properties were found to be anti-hypertensive, tranquilising, sedative, anti-convulsant to electric shock and it also had the ability to lower body temperature.

Jatamansone exhibited a tranquilising effect on a mouse and also on monkeys. In rabbits, it was found to impair biosynthesis of serotonin in the brain levels of 5-

hydroxytriptamine. The degeneration of the serotonin was unaffected. **It also** reduced hyperactivity, restlessness and aggressiveness in a study of hyper-kinetic children.

Jatamansone semicarbazone (a sesquiterpene ketone) was found to possess anti-estrogenic activity.

The Chemistry of Nardostachys Jatamansi

Nardostachys jatmansi is reported to have essential oils rich in coumarins and sesquiterpene. Major sesquiterpenes are Jatamansone and Valeroneas while the rest of sesquiterpenes are Jatamansol, jatamansic acid, dihydrojatamansin, nardosatchone Some minor contributors like jatamol A, jatamol B.[10], nardosinone, spirojatamol [11], jatamansinone, oroseolol, oroselone, valeranal, seselinnardostachyins, seychelane, seychellene, cuomarin and xynthogalin have also been reported as well as Alkaloids and actinidines.

In the main the chemical constituency of the root and the rhizome is coumarins and sesquiterpenes and it is these that are responsible most of the properties the essential oil. Sometimes however, it might be that source material for essential oil might be adulterated with Selinium vaginatum and selenium candollei (from the Apiacae genus), prior to distillation because the rhizomes look very alike.

The adulterated roots and oils may be sold unknowingly or be labelled correctly as *Bhutkeshi* or *Nakti jatamansi*, that is false jatamansi, predominately because of the lower commercial value, leading to far bigger profit margins.

Part 6 Clinical Evidence

As one might expect, we have India to thanks for the mainstay of the amassed clinical evidence into *Nardostachys jatamansi*. For the most part, as ever, these are experiments using alcoholic extractions rather than essential oils. Because we know that not every chemical constituents passes through distillation (most notable example would be that boswellic acid, the constituent causing such excitement in cancer trials is not found in the essential oil) that means that the chemical evidence found in these trials does not necessarily mean they will translate to aromatherapy. In the same way bear in mind that most of these trials are on animals or are in vitro studies. Whilst small mammals are used as the first stages of experimentation because they are evolutionarily so similar to humans, this does not necessarily mean that the medicine will translate to being effective medicine for us. Strangely of course, these trials to a certain extent are nothing more than validations of much of the traditional folk medicines of many, many centuries. I will warn you, though, if you thought we had left the sacrificial realms behind us, our rodent friends might argue otherwise. Oddly, there seem to be more in this book than in any of the others that went before.

We'll begin with an experiment done in 2008, to address the effects on the central nervous system, specifically to try to assess its antidepressant ability.

Antidepressant

Ethanoic extracts of 100, 200, 400mg/kg were given orally sweet little albino white mice. They were then subjected to Tail Suspension and Forced Swim tests. The mice which had been treated with the spikenard seemed to be significantly happier, exhibiting moods of similar quality than those that had been given two of the most often prescribed mood elevation drugs, Imipiramine and Sertraline.

These popular and successful drugs need to be monitored closely because, particularly in the first few weeks after having been prescribed to humans, there can be difficulties. These may present as behavioural changes and anxiety, panic attacks, sleeplessness, impulsive behaviour, aggressive and hostile outbursts. Patients can be agitated and very restlessness. They may become mentally or physically hyperactive or worse they may become even more depressed or even suicidal.

So spikenard was found to be as successful in elevating the mood as well as these drugs but without the locomotor activity (excessive grooming and scratching in mice for example, but in a human than might relate to wringing of hands, pacing the floor, smashing walls in frustration etc). Most interestingly they found that the spikenard was able inhibit expression of MAO –A and MAO-B throughout the body. (Remember we know it is the flavonoids that do this?)

MAO is short for *monamine oxidase*. Monamine oxidase inhibitors were some of the first synthetic antidepressants to be developed. The job of monamine oxidase is to break down norepinephrine, serotonin and dopamine, so the inhibitors prevented this breakdown meaning that concentrations of these mood elevation neurotransmitters were higher in the blood. These chemical versions of these drugs quickly went out of favour because side effects such as low blood pressure and lack of strength began to present themselves and it was found they didn't interact very well with some foods.

It is interesting to understand the functions of these strange genetic strains. They seem to have a very close relationship with mood but also aggressive behaviour. Here we discuss alleles which are genetic anomalies which occur at the same place on a chromosome. They can be dominant or recessive.

Ok the next bit feels complicated when you read it but it is easier to read on and come back…

In humans, there is a 30-base repeat sequence, repeated in one of several different numbers of times in the promoter region of the gene coding for MAO-A. These can be 2R (two repeats), 3R, 3.5R, 4R, and 5R variants of the repeat sequence. 3R and 4R variants are most common in Caucasians. In one study 3.5R and 4R variants were found to be more highly active than 3R or 5R. An association seems to exists between the 2R allele of the VNTR region of the gene and an increase in the likelihood of committing serious crime or violence has been found. (A variable number tandem repeat (or **VNTR**) is a location in a genome where a short nucleotide sequence is organized as a tandem repeat.)

Monoamine Oxidase A is associated with psychiatric disorders including antisocial behaviours. The oxidase is expressed through cardiac and neural cells and is modulated by stress through ischemia and inflammation.

Of most interest is the 3R mutation. It is associated with Brunner Syndrome, a condition which presents as a very low IQ, and problematic behaviours such as arson, hyper-sexuality and violence, as well as sleep disorders, and also autism.

It is also seen is Alzheimer's, aggression, panic disorder, bipolar affective disorder, major depressive disorder and attention deficit and hyperactivity disorders.

Elevated levels of the MOA in the 3R mutation are associated in 34% or people with Major Depressive Disorder. They can be associated with depressed suicides in men, sleep disorders and depression in men, and depression in females.

Interestingly though, maltreated children with high levels of the 3R mutation are less likely to develop antisocial behaviour in adulthood, but those who have lower levels are *more* likely to develop aggressive adulthood behaviours. Incredibly in one event, a murderer escaped the death penalty because his neurologist was able to show that his particular MAO mutation meant he was predisposed to being more violent toward women, although he was still sentenced to 32 years in gaol. (My English spelling *gaol* is so much more satisfying to write. Even I have to ask how that says *jail* though, I will concede!)

Now, I challenge you to read about MAO –B and not see Saturn medicine in every letter! Alzheimer's and Parkinson's diseases are both associated with elevated levels of MAO-B and scientists agree that it seems to be related to age and cognitive decline. It is also found to play a role in stress induced cardiac damage.

Inhibition of MAO-B in rats has prevented many age related biological changes such as optic nerve degeneration and has been shown to also prolong the rat's life by as much as 39%. There are many suggestions that MAO –B inhibitors may be a possible avenue of research to combat age related disease but this is a very controversial area. Regardless, since we have natural agent at our hands---it would be rude not to attempt it ourselves, don't you think?

Let's have a closer look at what that would do to mood now.

An alcoholic extract of Nardostachys jatamansi roots was given to some albino rats to assess the effects it had on levels of norepinephrine (NE), dopamine (DA), serotonin (5-HT), 5-hydroxyindoleacetic acid (5-HIAA), gamma-aminobutyric acid (GABA), and taurine in the brain, after 15 days of oral administration.

The effects were not immediate but at the end of the period a significant increase in the levels of NE, DA, 5-HT, 5-HIAA, and GABA was seen. The paper concludes "These data indicate that the alcoholic extract of the roots of N. jatamansi causes an overall increase in the levels of central monoamines and inhibitory amino acids."

Just in case you have not been able to keep up (because this book makes me dizzy, even if it doesn't make you) monoamines are crucial to cognition and arousal as well as keeping emotions level.

http://europepmc.org/abstract/med/8202559

Acetlycholinerase Inhibiting Activity

Around 50 different neurotransmitters have been identified in the brain. Acetylcholine (Ach) was the first to be characterized. It has a very significant presence and was recently determined as being essential for learning and memory. It has been a special target for research for almost two decades because deficiency among, other factors, maybe responsible for senile dementia and other degenerative cognitive disorders, including Alzheimer's Disease.

Alzheimer's Disease

One of the main hypotheses as to why Alzheimer's may occur is that senility seems to happen when there are tangles and lesions in the forebrain. It is proposed that this might be because of a cholinergic deficit.

Cholinergic means pertaining to Aceytlcholine, the neurotransmitters that, for the most part, fuel the parasympathetic nervous system. (We are talking about the part that is the braking mechanism for stress and looks after rest, recuperation and achieving homeostasis.) It seems as if these neurons become atrophied, thus causing a deficit.

Given that then, a great deal of study is being targeted into finding agents that can inhibit this AChE. Interestingly the only two drugs on the market authorised for use by the FDA, *rivastigmine* and *galantamine* are both plant derived too, (from daffodils and snowdrops) and so although they cannot cure the disease, only manage the symptoms, drug companies are looking to emulate this with other plant AChE inhibitors.

Acetlycholinerase (AChE) Inhibitors are found in conductive tissues such as nerves and muscles as well as motor and sensory fibres. For a cholinergic neuron to receive another impulse, ACh has to be be released from the ACh receptor. The active **site** of AChE comprises 2 subsites - the anionic **site** and the **esteratic** subsite. This is the part of a cholinesterase macromolecule that recognizes and binds to acetylcholine. If there is a lesion, then the message cannot get through. Reversible inhibitors settle into the esteratic site for short periods of time (seconds to minutes) and so are used to treat of a range of central nervous system diseases. In a 2007 trial several different herbs were tested and NJ was one of the successful ones to show mild acetylcholinerase activity.

In another study, several Indian Ayurvedic foods were tested. Although it was not the top performing (Indian gooseberry was) Nardostachys showed good AChE inhibiting potential and so has been proposed for further investigations towards therapy for Parkinson's, Alzheimer's and dementia patients.

As we've seen oxidation of cells is a concern and so the antioxidant properties of plants are of utmost interest to the men in white coats. In 2011 Hamdard University, (you will see these guys a lot. They have been busy!) wanted to investigate how giving some rats antioxidant supplementation might recover their learning abilities. The answer in this case was LOADS!

This time the ratties got a cocktail of crocetin, which is plant derived from saffron, as well as some of the natural mineral selenium. Well, if it is good enough for Adam after he was kicked out of the garden, and for Solomon in his Song of Songs we might expect there to be some pretty ace performance from a Spikenard and Saffron combination shouldn't we?

The rodent's passive avoidance stress test was improved as well as their performance in a maze. They remembered more, learned more and were more relaxed. And that my friends has made me go cold! I have goosebumps (I suppose that could be the Indian Gooseberry!). Three, four or maybe even five thousand years later and the cocktail comes back together again! It has been worth writing the book just to find that!!!!

http://link.springer.com/article/10.1007/s10072-011-0880-1

Hamdard University (bless 'em), India, 2006, and rats were treated with Nardstachys jatamansi for three weeks. On the 21st day they were then injected with 6-OHDA, a synthetic compound used by researchers to breakdown dopaminergic and noradrenergic neurons in the brain to simulate Parkinson's.

Each of the injuries or deficits caused by the drug was reversed by the jatamansi. (Importantly, they were dose dependently improved suggesting, that one drop of oil may not be enough in some cases of this kind of therapy.)

The 6-OHDA caused lesioning which was reversed by the NJ. The dose of 6-OHDA also decreased the amount of dopamine, but also the number of dopamine *receptors*. (So that means there were fewer opportunities for the already reduced amount of dopamine to grab onto.) Again NJ reversed this and restored these levels. The study concludes: "This study indicates that the extract of Jatamansi might be helpful in attenuating Parkinsonism."

http://www.sciencedirect.com/science/article/pii/S0091305 706000098

Dyskinesia

Now, I have to admit to having a rather obscene addiction to American dramas, most especially to The Good Wife. My favourite character is Louis Canning, played by Michael J Fox. The man's brilliance as a comedy actor is clear, as he manipulates the jury playing the sympathy vote for his involuntary facial twitches from tardive dyskinesia (although in reality, of course, he is affected by Parkinson's Disease which is also a spikenard friend). His latest shameless act of sending his crutches clattering to the floor during his opponent's moments of glory makes me howl, especially when Alicia accuses him of being "The Devil" and he looks like butter wouldn't melt. In reality though neither dyskinesia or Parkinson's are very much fun and I would love to see advances in the treatment that could help these people.

Reserpine-induced orofacial dyskinesia is an animal model of tardive dyskinesia where the rodent displays chewing movements and sticks their tongue out involuntarily. Here the rats were treated with alcoholic extracts on days one, three and five of the trial. The NJ significantly reduced the involuntary actions as well as cataplexy (where the patient experiences muscle weakness through strong emotions or laughter although they remain conscious).

The paper concludes that NJ:

"has potential value in the treatment of neuroleptic-induced orofacial dyskinesia and Parkinson's disease."

Learning and Memory

My poor old rats have been put through their paces for the cause of medicine, this time for learning, memory and cognition.

I'll draw several trials together for brevity.

Firstly they were tested in an Elevated Plus Maze, which tests anxiety by watching their aversion to bright open spaces. Since they naturally prefer to be hidden behind something tall and in a dark place, anxiety reduction is determined by how much more time they spend in the open arms of the maze.

They were also subjected to the Passive Avoidance Paradigm, by placing the animal into a brightly lit box. Since they prefer the safety of darkness, the rodent will naturally try to find ways to get out of the brightness. When they get to the darkness however they receive a small electric shock teaching them that there are negative consequences to being in that space. Consequently they try to learn and remember new exit routes to escape their fear.

Both young and old mice were given 8 successive days treatment of three doses (50, 100, and 200 mg/kg, p.o.) of an ethanolic extract of N. jatamansi. (P.O. by the way means orally.) The largest dose of N.J significantly improved the learning and memory in the younger mice, but it also reversed the amnesia induced by diazepam and scopolamine. What's more, it also reversed aging-induced amnesia that can be ascribed to the natural aging of the mice... (Here, I would recommend you have a quick check back to Rose Goddess Medicine and have a look at the notes on schapolamine there too) Because there was a reversal seen in the scopolamine-induced amnesia, it could be that the memory improvement might have happened because of a facilitation of cholinergic transmission in the brain.

Regardless of the mechanism, *N. jatamansi* may prove to be useful in the treatment of dementia seen in elderly persons. Again, there is a suspicion that the actions may come from antioxidant properties.

http://online.liebertpub.com/doi/abs/10.1089/jmf.2006.9.11 3

Chronic fatigue Syndrome

India 2008, a model of Chronic Fatigue was used to assess NJ anti-oxidant capabilities. Rats were put into three groups this time. One was a standard control group, one being treated with ginseng, also as a control and our NJ.

The rats were forced to swim for 15 minutes a day, for twenty one consecutive days. In the control groups, they quickly started to exhibit despair behaviour and anxiety. This did not happen in the NJ rats.

Their locomotor activity – them moving from one place to another- decreased in the control groups. Not so with the spikenard.

When they were sacrificed and analysed the oxidant levels had gone through the roof, but the NJ had reduced lipid peroxidation, nitrites and levels of catalyse. (Now that last sentence might seem like I was speaking Welsh again, but hold your nerve till we get to the heart medicine section where we will cover that in a bit more detail.)

http://www.sciencedirect.com/science/article/pii/S0166432 809002216

http://www.ncbi.nlm.nih.gov/pmc/articles/PMC3371456/

These following trials also all proved anti-oxidant abilities through various convoluted and complicated means! Feel free to read and translate if you so desire.

http://www.ncbi.nlm.nih.gov/pubmed/24632018

http://www.ncbi.nlm.nih.gov/pubmed/23573115

Anticonvulsant

Florida 2004, Nardostachys jatamansi increased the seizure threshold in rats which had been treated with electric shocks.

Unfortunately it was not as effective to those which had seizures induced by pentylenetetrazole.

This helps us to identify a little more about what may be happening with the spikenard action. Pentylenetetrazole is used as an assay because it excites gaba receptors. This drug is chosen because its effects emulate the "petit-mal" seizures of humans where the electrical shocks are more similar to those previously known as "grand mal" now more recently referred to as tonic clonic seizures.

In these tonic-clonic seizures the body stiffens. The patient tends to cry or groan as air is forced past the vocal. The tonic phase is when they fall to the ground. As the clonic phase begins, limbs jerk in strong, rhythmic movements. A petit mal attack will make the person temporarily "absent"and experience a temporary loss of consciousness.

In short then, the spikenard had far better effects with the dramatic shaking version of epilepsy which, actually, given its effects on tremors, is exactly what we might expect to see.

http://www.sciencedirect.com/science/article/pii/S0378874 10500423X

So we have seen that the mice learn better, and I have to admit to wanting to raid some labs and open some electrocuted cages for these poor oppressed rodents, but this next trial made me put the crow bar down.

Here, scientists wanted to examine how we learn in stressful environments (Clearly this is a factor behind the horrors of PTSD for example.)

So the trial is to establish to what extent NJ protects against impairments that chronic stress causes in spatial learning and memory. This time, rats were exposed to 21 days of chronic restraint stress. They simultaneously received either 100 mg or 200 mg/kg of NJE (The E is extract.). Then their memories were tested by putting them into in a partially-baited eight arm radial maze.

Those animals which had been treated with the larger dose of spikenard had learning curves similar to the unstressed animals that had been used as control subjects. They made significantly more correct choices (38%) and fewer memory errors (53%, $P < 0.01$) when they were tested on the eighth day of training compared to untreated, stressed animals. (The effects of them receiving the larger dose were significantly better).

What's more, after ten days, they were racking up scores far more impressively than the untreated controls. They made significantly higher correct choices (31%, $P <$ 0.001) than untreated animals when they were given a memory retention test. So the scientists proposed that spikenard probably has a protective effect of stress-induced impairments in hippocampus-dependent learning and memory behaviour in rats. For me though, I can't help but think that pitta energy and rhaktu dhatu are raised by too much study and spikenard helps to reduce that internal bodily heat. It amounts to the same thing, doesn't it?

http://jnsbm.org/article.asp?issn=0976-9668;year=2012;volume=3;issue=2;spage=125;epage=132;aulast=Karkada

Stress

Four groups of rats were stressed for four hours by being placed in temperatures of 4 degrees centigrade. Then they were sacrificed (how very Saturnic, they were sent to a cold place to suffer and then they were sent to Mme. La Guillotine). They were assessed in many different ways to compare the effects NJ had had on their bodies alongside those rats that had had no herbal treatment.

Those with no treatment had gastric ulcerations, but those treated with NJ had been inhibited. The spikenard group had reduced adrenal and splenic weights and also decreased levels of ascorbic acid in the adrenals (ascorbic acid/vitamin C release is a precursor to cortisol release in the adrenals). They had significantly reduced levels of lipid peroxidations (where free radicals steal electrons from the cells and cause damage leading to red cell rupture) and decreased levels of nitric oxide. These actions may be due to spikenard's antioxidant action.

Heart Function

A 2007 study by the University of Madras in Tamil Nado wanted to investigate the effects of jatamansi on cardiac cells that have been put under pressure. Two groups of albino rats, one treated for seven days prior to cardiac injury with an oral dose of jatamansi.

Cardiac injury was induced by a single dose of doxorubicin, an antibiotic usually used to treat leukaemia and other types of cancer.

Heart function changes mainly because the altered lipid metabolism changes the cardiac cell membranes. The doxopubicin induced raised levels of cholesterol, triglycerides, free fatty acids and phospholipids as well as significantly raising levels of lipoproteins. In all cases, the NJ rats were protected against these changes, again potentially because if the anti-lipid peroxidative properties.

Heart NO

Nitric oxide plays a large part in my book on bronchitis. I'm going to copy a section across to here for you:

In 1992, Nitric Oxide was named Molecule of The Year by the journal *Science* but it took another 6 years for the scientists who had made the discoveries surrounding it, to be awarded the Nobel Prize for Chemistry. Three parties, Robert F. Furchgott, PhD, Louis J. Ignarro, PhD, and Ferid Murad, MD, PhD were jointly awarded the 1998 prize for their work surrounding the molecule.

Nitric oxide is a neutrotransmitter, (the job of a neurotransmitter is to relay signals from the nervous system to the physiology of the body). It is one of the few neurotransmitters in the body that is a gas. It is found in the tissues of every cell and so there is nowhere in our system that is more than one micron away from a supply of it. Its state as a gas means it can move through the body at a startling speed, far faster than many other neurotransmitters.

Its job, very simplistically speaking, is to smooth tissues. It plays a massive part in the cardiovascular and nervous systems. It is now also understood to play a fundamental part in immunity. It is found in the endothelial tissues (the lining) of each cell and it signals vascular smooth cells to relax so vasodilation can take place. Veins and arteries are filled with this relaxant gas and as Nitric Oxide (NO) is activated, it triggers blood vessels to open, allowing parts of the body to be better supplied with circulation.

It is released into our systems at times of pleasure. The best example of how it works is in sexual function. When a man is pleasured, nitric oxide floods through his system allowing blood to flow more freely and effectively to his penis, engorging it and causing an erection. The same happens to a woman when her clitoris is stimulated, but that, clearly, is harder to see!

In February 2015, spikenard oil was placed into cultures with phosphorescent dye to watch how Nitric oxide was triggered.

Their findings suggested that the oil was able to control vascular dilatation, and this was mediated by its ability to trigger NO production.

http://www.ncbi.nlm.nih.gov/pubmed/25643147

http://www.ingentaconnect.com/content/govi/pharmaz/2007/00000062/00000005/art00013

Rat Ischaemia

Ischaemia is inadequate blood supply to an organ or part of the body, especially the heart muscles. A trial from Hamdad University India, proved that protected rat brains from ischaemia.

Liver damage

Hamdard University 2002 showed that also spikenard protected rats against liver damage.

http://www.sciencedirect.com/science/article/pii/S0378874199001531

Insomnia

I do love to find a clinical trial that comes from complementary therapy rather than from universities and hospitals, because they seem to have so much more of a holistic bias. The language is softer and far more engaging to read.

This sleep study is from an Indian Ayurvedic hospital and University as well as an old people's home in Kerala.

It opens with the shocking statement that in 2004 the World Health Organisation estimated the burden of the fact that between 30-35% of people suffer from insomnia costs the global economy 3.6 million absent work days every year.

The trial separates primary insomnia from secondary insomnia which is sleeplessness due to some kind of other disorder, injury, emotional or physical disorder. So primary insomnia, then, is simply being unable to sleep for no apparent reason.

To be included into the trial the 34 participants all matched the criteria:

- They had been suffering insomnia up to 5 years duration
- They could be of either sex, but were aged between 15 and 45 years
- And they also complained of *Angamarda* (bodyache), *Shirogaurava* (heaviness in the head), *Jrumbha* (yawning), *Jadyata* (inactivity), *Glani* (exhaustion), *Bhrama* (giddiness), *Apakti* (indigestion).

So, here the patients were treated with two herbal powders, both of which are interesting to us. The first is *Valeriana wallichii*, known as *Tagara* in local medicine and we also see our *Nardostachys grandiflora*. They were given a 4g dose with milk three times a day.

Actually, Tagara was the more efficient of the two herbs but spikenard fared well enough for us to be impressed.

In total 34 patients were studied in two groups; only 30 patients completed the course of treatment (15 in each).

So how did the insomnia present itself? I'm leaving the Ayurvedic terms in because sometimes there is no direct translation and so there is a sense of something, rather than an actual word we might recognise. So, these are closest translations.

Of 34 patients, specific causative factors of *Anidra* (insomnia) were felt to be *chinta* (excessive thinking), which was observed in a massive 85.29% of the patients

- 64.71% felt it was anxiety (*udvega*). Sadly, 29.41% felt their sleeplessness was probably down to depression (*vishada*), and 38.23% said specifically they were worrying about family problems.
- 73.52% found it very difficult to get to sleep at night
- 52.94% described having disturbed sleep.
- 47.05% felt that it disturbed their routine work, day to day.

The associated symptoms of a bad night's sleep were reported as

Shirogaurava (heaviness in the head) in 64.70% of the group

61.76% described symptoms of *Angamarda* (aching body).

47.05% described being fatigued (*Shrama*).

44.11% reported having *Klama* (mental fatigue) and Shirashula (shooting pains in the head)

Other complaints were:

- *Glani* (exhaustion) in 41.17%,
- *Aruchi* (distaste) in 38.23%
- *Apakti* (indigestion) 35.29%
- *Jrumbha* (yawning) 35.29%
- *Jadyata* (inactivity) and *Tandra* (stupor) in 29.41% each
- *Bhrama* (giddiness) in 23.52% of patients.

Not a pretty picture. Actually, it is a quite a miserable one really, isn't it, given that some of these people had been suffering for up to five years.

So, they were given a treatment of herbal powders to use for a month.

The Tagara group showed a significant improvement in the duration of their sleep by 55.17%. 76.00% had found it easier to get to sleep and the reduction in disturbances of their sleep dropped by 69.58%. The improvement in the disturbances in their routine work was a massive 73.95%

The Jatamansi group was in second place but that certainly does not detract from its most impressive results. It provided a 61.34% improvement in the initiation of sleep, a 48.25% enhancement in the duration of sleep. The disturbance in every day routine works dropped by 43.85%, and a 53.08% decrease was seen in disturbed sleep.

Jatamansi gave significant relief in:

- *Angamarda* (aching body) 39.16%
- *Shirogaurava* (heavy head) 41.87%
- *Shirashoola* (head pain) 66.67%
- *Jrumbha* (yawning) 50.00%
- *Aruchi* (distaste) 58.75%
- *Shrama* (fatigue) 45.11%
- *Klama* (mental fatigue) 56.00%

Because I am a generous Buy-one-Get-One Free kinda gal... here's the wallichii results.

Tagara provided significant relief in

- *Angamarda* (aching body) 78.33% improvement
- *Shirogaurava* (heavy head) 72.60%
- *Shirashoola* (pains in the head) 55.83%
- *Jrumbha* (yawning) 26.41%
- *Glani* (exhaustion) 36.79%
- *Bhrama* (giddiness) 86.02%
- *Shrama* (80.45%) and *Klama* (physical and mental fatigue) 83.33%

I have noticed that Oshadhi sell a wallichi essential oil and that is going to be my next shopping list treat.

http://www.ncbi.nlm.nih.gov/pmc/articles/PMC4687238/

PCOS

August 2015, Kerala, and scientists are potentially changing the face of women's medicine by isolating which plants might be able to help alleviate the growing problem of Poly Cystic Ovarian Syndrome.

They completed a RIKILT yeast Androgen bioassay which measures levels of androgen in urine. In this particular experiment rats had PCOS induced by the use of estradion valerate.

Various plants were tested but Nardostachys proved to be the most effective in reversing the androgenic effects.

Interestingly the other plant which achieved equally impressive results was Tribulus terrestris, not an essential oil we use but I am sure that you have heard of its herbal prowess for improving male sexuality...this is Horny Goat Weed.

So this gives me pause, really, because how does that work? The paper cites both NJ and TT as having antiandrogenic properties. Anti-androgens are popular in orthodox medicine for treating any number of complaints from prostate problems, to seborrhoea and acne, and hyper sexuality. That is they are used to *diminish* libido, and yet Tribulus terratis is probably the world's biggest selling sexuality booster. So I am not sure. It is a quandary. Nevertheless the trial concludes with the statement "NJ and TT extract treatment normalized estrous cyclicity and steroidal hormonal levels and regularized ovarian follicular growth."

So we can say that Nardostachys jatamansi has anti-androgenic properties and as such it should be indicated for PCOS because it brings the estrogen levels into balance, it settles the hormonal levels down and it calms the growth of the ovarian follicles.

Pancreatitis

Acute pancreatitis affects about 300 people per million a year.

Symptoms of the disease include

- Upper abdominal pain that radiates into the back. This can be aggravated by eating, especially foods high in fat
- Swollen and tender abdomen
- Nausea and vomiting
- Fever
- Increased heart rate

Pancreatic damage occurs because the pancreatic enzymes are triggered before food reaches the small intestine and so they begin attacking the pancreas.

Acute pancreatitis is a sudden pain that can lead to discomfort for a short amount of time. It can range from mildly uncomfortable to being a life threatening disease. It is relatively easy to treat and recovery is usually fast, however in some cases pancreatitis can cause the gland to bleed, cause tissue damage or the formation of cysts. It can also cause damage to the lungs, heart and kidneys. When it gets to this point, patients will be admitted to hospital.

About one in ten occurrences of acute pancreatitis is deemed to be severe and about a third of all deaths associated with acute pancreatitis are associated with the occurring lung injury.

Experts from School of Oriental Medicine, Wonkwang University, Iksan, Jeonbuk, South Korea wanted to see if Nardostachys jatamansi might hold some answers to treating these sad and painful cases. Their 2010 investigations focused on dealing with mild cases of acute pancreatitis.

They induced pancreatitis in rats using cerulean, which is a ten amino acid peptide that stimulates digestive and smooth muscle.

The rats were split into two groups, a pre treatment group and a post treatment group.

In the pretreatment group, N. jatamansi was given orally to the mice at 10 and 20 mg/kg for 5 days, and then our rodent heros were intraperitoneally injected with the cerulean, every hour for 6 hours.

In the post treatment group, cerulein was injected hourly for 6 hours, and then N. jatamansi was given at 1, 3, and 5 hours after the first cerulein injection.

Blood samples were taken 6 hours later to assess the serum amylase (the enzyme that helps to us to digest carbohydrates, the lipase (breaks down fats to fatty acids), and the cytokine levels (secreted by the immune system to affect other cells) .

Sadly, then, the poor old pancreatic rodents had their tiny lungs and pancreases removed for analysis.

Amazingly there had been a reduction to the pancreatic oedema, the neutrophil infiltration (while blood cell count), serum amylase and lipase levels, serum cytokine levels, and messenger RNA expressions of inflammatory mediators. In English that means that the spikenard reduced the pancreatic swelling and prevented the messengers being sent to the lung, which would inflame and damage it. Thus spikenard reduced the effects of the pancreatitis and protected the lung from damage.

http://www.ncbi.nlm.nih.gov/pubmed/22831975

Then, in 2012, they wanted to build on these findings at was and stretched the tests to focus on severe acute pancreatitis. Rats again, this time they had pancreatitis induced by a diet that was deficient in choline and then supplemented by an amino acid called ethionine. They were then give NJ, in powdered form dissolved into saline for seven days.

The rats were sacrificed and the results collated. It was found that the pancreatitis had severely affected the tissues of the pancreas and that lipase and amylase had been hyper-stimulated, sending inflammatory markers from the organ. But the rats treated with the NJ showed a different story. The herb had attenuated the release of the interleukin 1 & 6 (inflammatory markers) and the Tumour Necrosis Factor. It had stopped the enzyme damage, as well as the digestive damage, and so researchers were able to ascertain that it was the digestive reaction that had given protection to the pancreas. A later study done in South Korea, last year, pinpointed that the active constituent responsible for the anti-inflammatory properties was most likely desoxo-narchinol-A

http://www.ncbi.nlm.nih.gov/pubmed/23181131

Fungitoxic

A very useful piece of research if you have found your way to the book by means of wanted to help respiratory conditions, in particular COPD which is exacerbated by moulds and fungus.

A 1995 by University of Gorakhpur proved that Nardostachys jatamansi completely wiped out samples of Aspergillus flavus, Aspergillus niger, and Fusarium oxysporum at a concentration of 1.0×10^3 µL/L

http://cat.inist.fr/?aModele=afficheN&cpsidt=3529058

It seems to me the only remaining question mark now is….

Hair Care

In *Pharmacographica Indica: A History of the Principal Drugs of Vegetable Origin, Met with in British India,* (1890) William Dymock revealed the main Indian use of the drug was making hairwashes and ointments popularly thought to promote growth and blackness of the hair. We know the Corinthians used it to paint their eyebrows on more thickly and Avicenna says it will make the eyelashes fuller. But can it really be true that a root can make your hair grow…? I'm suspicious because eating my crusts never made my hair curl and I believed that one for nearly forty years! I'll not be so easily persuaded again.

Here, several different natural products including jatamansi, coffee and henna were tested to see how effective they were in colouring the hair. The results showed the spikenard is most certainly able to deepen the blackness of hair.

http://www.ncbi.nlm.nih.gov/pubmed/26130937

CavinKare Research Centre in Chennai then wanted to know if NJ was able to influence hair *growth* too. This is an interesting study because they put the root through fractional distillation and isolated the various constituents to see which bits were creating the magic.

This time our furry friends became unfurry, thanks to some depilatory cream, were washed clean and then treated with a solution of either Jatamansi or Minoxidil which is a hypertensive drug reputed to make your hair grow and then, finally there was a control of no treatment.

Surprisingly there seemed to be no extra growth for the Minoxidil, but the components of Nardin and jatamasic acid both reduced hair growth time. To me though, that just says that your hair grows faster...not that it makes it grow. If that makes sense? Since CavinCare makes shampoos though, that is still worthwhile data for them.

http://www.ncbi.nlm.nih.gov/pmc/articles/PMC3113354/

But we can build on that thanks to a 2009 study Bharati Vidyapeeth's College of Pharmacy, in Navi-Mumbai. They too wanted to compare results with minoxidil, but this time they used a tresses cocktail.

Theirs was *Eclipta alba Hassk* also known as False Daisy, 10%, *Hibiscus rosa sinensis Linn* of Chinese Hibiscus 10 % and Nardostachys jatamansi in a herbal oil. (No species was given for the carrier.)

The growing time of the hair was *halved!* Quantitative analysis of hair growth after the treatment with the oil blend showed a greater number of hair follicles in the anagenic phase. This is where the follicle splits and divides. The root of the hair divides rapidly thus adding to the shaft. Normally this phase means that hair would grow 1cm every 28 days. The miracle oil then, meant that cm was shortened to just 14 days.

Now...yes I am happier with that!

http://sphinxsai.com/PTVOL4/pdf_vol4/PT=46%20(1251-1254).pdf

Cancer

This is the section I hate writing the most, but for the sake of completeness it needs to be in. Please though, understand this. Essential oils make cells grow. This book shows this not least in the hair research, it grew twice as fast. We certainly don't want to do that to a cancer cell. Also I don't care what the MLM's tell you there is no essential oil proven to be a cure for cancer. Frankincense might be a medicine of the future but it does boswellic acid does not pass through distillation. Often when these essential oils are tested in blood rather than simply in a petri dish they bubble up and lose their efficacy. The journey from establishing an active constituent to making it a drug that can be used on actual people as a licenced medicine is long, arduous and not our business. Please, leave treating cancer to the experts.

That said, it is interesting to see where the medicines may come from so let's see what Nardostachys jatamansi is able to do.

Extracts taken from the whole jatamansi plant showed selective cytotoxicity against certain lines of prostate and colon cancers.

http://www.ncbi.nlm.nih.gov/pubmed/25971678

A 95% alcoholic extract (ACE) was tested on human cancer cell lines at 10, 30 and 100 µg/ml respectively.

It showed percent growth inhibition of 11, 42 and 71 % against lung cancer hells

10, 37 and 80 % against liver (Hep-2),

17, 29 and 73 % ovarian cancer

4, 43 and 90 % against prostate (PC-3)

The results revealed that extracts of *N. jatamansi* could decrease the survival rate of four different human cancer cell lines in a dose- and time-dependent manner. Cell proliferation was significantly inhibited by ACE and from the first day of culture.

It was also found that it was effective against sarcoma.

http://www.omicsgroup.org/journals/in-vitro-and-in-vivo-biological-activities-of-nardostachys-jatamansi-roots.pdf-2167-0412.1000142.php?aid=21950

Nardostachys jatamansi diethyl ether was effective against breast carcinoma.

http://www.ncbi.nlm.nih.gov/pubmed/25886964

Modulates radiation

Let's end on a good note, and paradoxically this one also pertains to cancer. It is beautiful and could potentially revolutionise the face of medicine. One of the most aggressive weapons we have against cancer is radiation. Thank Goddess for it, but the side effects of the treatment can be horrible. In the first couple of days there can be vomiting, diarrhoea and nausea, but then this becomes more complex as the radiation begins to attack the bone marrow and spleen causing blood problems. This is termed haematopoietic syndrome. This is usually a side effect of having undergone whole body irradiation, and the splenic damage is often a factor in mortality.

Here rats were treated with a dose of alcoholic extract of spikenard once a day for fifteen days before the irradiation and for fifteen days after it. Blood samples were taken and at the end of the experiment the mice were sacrificed.

The blood tests showed that the rats in the control group had significantly impaired levels of haemoglobin, erythrocytes, leukocytes, the packed cell volume and the platelet count. These bone marrow cells are vital to life and so any damage will be irreversible and will significantly impact on health.

The picture was markedly different in those lucky rats who had been treated with the spikenard extract. Their sickness and diarrhoea levels were less. All of their red, white blood cell levels, their haemoglobin, packed cell count and bone marrow counts were high...in fact almost as high as if they had not even had the radiation! Their little bodies had been completely protected meaning that their mortality levels would have been much lover...had they not been sacrificed to the guillotine for the sake of our science.

http://www.ncbi.nlm.nih.gov/pubmed/23716877

A 2012 study showed that these beneficial effects on the bone marrow are most likely due to its anti-oxidant prowess.

http://www.ncbi.nlm.nih.gov/pubmed/23905085

I still very much stand by the statement of no essential oils on the body in treatment, and I will keep on believing that until the scientists tell us otherwise, but inhalation of spikenard before and after radiation treatment...I think it has got to be a good recommendation.

And without a shade of irony now, I am going to suggest we take a moment to say thank you. Thank you to all these rodents who have gone to their Saturnic deaths in the name of science for our better lives. Their sacrifices will truly bring about better health. More, a thank you to the Great Mother for medicine in the plants and thank you to all these scientists who are working tirelessly to find these cures.

So we understand what the men in the white coats think of our root. We know how Ayurveda uses it. We have an understanding of how it was used in history, but how do other aromatherapists use it, I wondered.

Part 7 Clinical Recommendations from Other Authorities
I thought it would be interesting for you to read how other therapists use spikenard in their practices. I am so grateful to these people for sharing their knowledge with us. I deliberately chose people who had very specialist knowledge in their areas as a means to introduce some other fabulous authorities to you. Please do take the time to visit them on facebook, read their books and take a peek at their websites. To me, these are some of the most gifted people in their fields. These are the people I would want to learn from. They hail

from every corner of the Earth: from England, Germany, Holland, Hungary, Hong Kong and USA.

As the pieces they had written started to trickle into my email I felt so very blessed to be surrounded and supported by these people. Their tales are magical, of genuine healing for people and creatures when they have been in crisis. None of us have seen each other's work until I put it all together. It is remarkable how the same knowledge translates in so many different ways.

Their gifts of writing give spikenard a newly enigmatic dimension and whilst their therapy in essence is the same as mine, their language of healing makes the therapy take flight.

The Phoenix is very happy with the beautiful sounds and fragrances of this section!

Gergely Hollódi

Gergely and I started chatting on theInternational Federation ofAromatherapists's (IFPA) forum one day, when a group of us were trying to fathom out a way to treat a particularly puzzling patient case. It soon became clear were kindred neuroscience junkies.

I sent him some of the books I had written, because Amazon is not available in Hungary. A few days later he asked me to write for his Hungarian aromatherapy magazine Aromatika.hu. I promise you there is no buzz in the world like seeing your work in Hungarian when Gergely has finished with it because he makes it look glorious with the wonderfully surprising pictures he adds.

I think the universe wanted us to meet. We have a pattern. It goes like this Gergely says please will you write about this? I go yes, and think what on Earth am I going to write? I hit the books and get sucked into a vortex of research I would not have found otherwise and another book is born. Both the Rose and Clary Sage books are thanks to his inspiration.

This is a man for whom nothing seems too much trouble. He always has something inspiring or comforting to say and the world of aromatherapy is lucky to have him. I am lucky to count him as my friend.

Spikenard, the guttural voice – Gergely Hollódi

Spikenard or Nard for me is one of the most mysterious essential oils. When I first smelt it I had controversial feelings. I have never experienced such a scent. On the one hand I had a shimmering feeling running up and down my spine, on the other hand I felt a deeply relaxing swing in my brain. One can immediately feel the slightly earthy while balsamic, warm, woody, bittersweet and slightly peat-reminding notes of this oil. This is not surprising, taking into consideration that the essential oil is obtained from the slender rootlet-covered rhizomes of the plant.

Nard has a captivating aroma, almost pinning me to Earth, grounding yet wisely elevating spiritually. It immediately rings tones of throat singing in my ears. Mongolian throat singing is something which tells us so much about one's inner voice manifested through the vocal chords emerging from deep down the lungs. And indeed, when I inhale the Spikenard oil it goes down deep. No, not the deep Hyssop would go. It doesn't stop at the farthest niche of the lungs but goes deeper, down to my legs and further. Like roots... So the more I smell the oil the more the singing goes on with the resonating guttural voice.

Nard; knowing it was one of a secret and sacred ingredients in ointments and incenses for at least three world religions always adds to its mystic qualities to me. One of my best natural perfumery base combinations is Nard with Somali deep orange colored Myrrh. Adding Jasmine excelerates the synergy... It smells sweetish-spicy but with a powerful note that I can imagine to emit from a traveling robe of a frigate captain just returning to Europe from farther worlds at the dawn of colonization.

Nard from another point of view, and my experience is not appealing to many. Some say they don't like the smell, some might feel scared. But all agree that it is a deep aroma that goes down all the way. One of my former students when smelt Nard for the first time called me a few days after. She said first she was no friends with the oil but she had dreams the following nights. She needed to admit that the oil was so powerful that she had to admit that some feelings that were locked for many years have opened up and she released. No wonder that many of us aromatherapists use this oil for nervous conditions, calming. I have heard of people who use this oil in palliative care because it helps the terminally ill to come to peace with the world.

Nard indeed, is a powerful and mysterious yet multi-faced substance that when used at the right place and time can aid us humans through troubled times. For me it always lingers around like the voice of a Mongolian throat singer's lullaby.

Kelly Holland Azzarro

You know how, sometimes, you just click with someone? That is how it is with Kelly and me. She gets my sense of humour and she works as fast as I do! It is a recipe for success.

Usually it is I who is the spectre at the feast, lurking in the background, but this time it had been Kelly. When I write for the NAHA magazine, normally the gorgeous Sharon Falsetto of Sedona Aromatherapy edits my work, but quietly in the background (sighing in dismay at my long winded prose, I am sure) was Kelly also putting great lines through my work.

My interest was piqued the second she contacted me on Facebook because I had no idea there were so many people interested in aromatherapy for animals. I often get asked about it, but would not know where to start. Kelly is magical with these creatures and when you read her posts you can see she is like a modern day Dr Doolittle. They are just enchanting to read.

Animal Aromatherapy by Kelly Holland Azzaro RA, CCAP, CBFP, LMT

Spikenard for Fear-based Issues

I have used spikenard essential oils for animals that have suffered from a past trauma that has contributed to them being stuck in a fear-based state that would manifest in a variety of different symptoms including: chronic anxiousness, separation anxiety, reactive to loud noises and changes in routine, and with most of the animals that have been abused or traumatized they may also develop a hypersensitivity or guarded reaction to touch. Some animals even carry around this fear as in a constant state of post-traumatic stress disorder.

Hypersensitivity to touch can manifest from several issues, mostly due to a past injury or trauma (physical or emotional), as well as after a surgery when the Meridian energetics may be stagnant. This is often seen in animals that have been abused. The animal may show signs of guarding of the localized area (physical trauma/post-surgery/injury) and quiver or be jumpy when touched. You may also notice that they roll a lot in an attempt to 'shake-off' the excess energy/stagnation, etc.

Using acupressure and aromatherapy (as well as Bach Flower essences) all of which will help to reduce this type of sensitivity/reaction.

The use of spikenard via inhalation and in a topical application diluted in a carrier base can be quite effective in restoring your animal's sense of calm and well-being. 1 drop of essential on a tissue for direct inhalation as needed, or place 2-4 drops of spikenard essential oil into 1 oz. of carrier base (aloe vera gel or jojoba) applied topically to the mid chest area as needed. A mist spray may also be made with diluted distilled water (2 oz.) and lavender (*Lavandula angustifolia*) hydrosol (2 oz.) and a few drops of spikenard essential oil for misting through the animal's fur or sprayed near their bedding. If irritation occurs discontinue use.

Safety cautions: avoid use of essential oils with cats and birds and do not diffuse essential oils near fish and reptile or small mammal's habitats.

Kelly Holland Azzaro, RA, CCAP, CBFP, LMT, is a Registered Aromatherapist, Certified Clinical Aromatherapy Practitioner,

Certified Bach Flower Practitioner, Licensed Massage Therapist, Reiki Practitioner, Past Vice President (NAHA), Past President of NAHA and current Public Relations, Journal Manger and Co-Editor of NAHA (National Association for Holistic Aromatherapy).

Kelly has over 20 years professional experience and educational training in Aromatherapy and Massage Therapy. She also has specialized training in Canine and Equine Acupressure-Massage Therapies, Intuitive Animal Communication, Crystal-Gemstone Therapy, Reiki, Aromatherapy and Flower Essence Therapy for people and their animal friends.

Kelly is approved by the National Certification Board of Therapeutic Massage and Bodywork (NCBTMB) as a Continuing Education Approved Provider, and her (300+hr) Animal Aromatherapy Practitioner Certification Course(sm) meets the NAHA Standards of Education requirements. Kelly is the Founder and Director of The Holistic Animal Association Network.

Kelly, and her husband Marco a Licensed Acupuncturist and Qigong Practitioner/Instructor have a Holistic Healing Center where they work together as a team to educate and empower others through holistic services, education and support.

URL: ashitherapy.com | www.holisticanimalassociation.com

Madeleine Kerkhof-Knapp Hayes

Madeleine and I are great Facebook friends and I am excited that our paths will probably cross several times this year, but most certainly when we both speak at the NAHA conference in Utah in October.

Madeleine is one of life's gentle people. Good people. Someone I wish was I could be like. She is the leading authority in using aromatherapy for palliative care and you must please read her book. It is so detailed and yet easy to read. It has opened doors to a new way for nurses and doctors to care for their patients to ensure they have the best death that they can. I think you will love the way she writes.

Spikenard & Sensitivity by Madeleine Kerkhof-Knapp Hayes

In my time as a nurse specialized in complementary aromatherapy, I have grown fond of spikenard through the years. I never thought much of the – to me – heavy and earthy fragrance until I blended it with the finest essential oils of neroli, rose CO_2 extract and Angelica seed oil. In diffusion this gives me a very comforting, calming and consoling atmosphere when I need it, especially in times of grief and sadness.

Case – Madeleine: sleepless

In busy periods I tend to mull over the day quite extensively. Instead of picking a suitable time, my mind likes to play tricks with me in the middle of the night. I knew spikenard could be extremely calming. I read some Indian research on that. I tried Nepalese spikenard in combination with lavender, mandarin, neroli and frankincense because I used to sleep very restlessly. I did like the blend, but somehow it just wasn't doing it for me. Nepalese spikenard has a pale to dark greenish colour. On its own the fragrance is earthy and makes me think of walking through a dewed autumn forest.

Of course I knew that there was Indian spikenard as well. For quite some years it was hard to find, but recently I received some from a small distillers near Mumbai. What a revelation this has been! It has a rich brown colour, much like maple syrup, and its fragrance is just amazing. It is earthy, but with a depth that I never smelled before. It has layers of fragrance that develop one by one. When I first smelled it, the oil instantly grounded me and almost forced me to dive deep into myself and just feel . I felt protected, rooted yet in touch with all of me: body, heart, head and soul. There was a great sense of peace flowing gently through all of my being. When I added that to my blend instead of the Nepalese oil, it made a great difference. I use it in an Aromapatch® and that is a very good way of using essential oils at night. I feel much more calm at night and sleep through the night much more often.

Since spikenard is given to help people who are highly sensitive, I used it in a blend for a beautiful lady in the terminal stage of her life (this case is in my book).

Case – Bea: highly sensitive

In September 2012 I received a phone call from nurse Ina from the hospice Bethlehem in Nijmegen, the Netherlands. She wanted to talk to me about Bea, a former nurse and who was now nearing the end of her journey here on earth. She had lung cancer and suffered from severe dyspnoea.

However, Bea also had another problem. She was extremely sensitive to the perception and energy of others around her. The problem was that the highly empathetic woman with her warm heart could barely shield herself from the backpack full of problems of well-intentioned caregivers, and even a foot massage became too much. Bea shut down, both literally and figuratively. The tightness she felt in her chest – at least this is what Ina said – was typical of this. It was like she was "hardly breathing in complete silence". Bea told Ina that the overwhelming amount of impressions from others really hindered her to open up her mind to the passing away.

That is why, after consulting with Bea, Ina contacted me to see in what way we could use aromas to provide support. Bea would benefit most from oils that could help her get air and space, both in physical and in emotional and spiritual sense. Together we made a selection from the oils available in the hospice to be used during the first few hours after their request for help, which included the clear and fresh Scots pine, fragrant and deeply calming olibanum CO2, and a gentle and light "high altitude" lavender.

Bea said that the pine immediately opened up her lungs and that she experienced a sensation of more space. The olibanum gave her a quiet, soft and dreamy expression. She thought the lavender was just "beautiful!". Therefore, Ina prepared an inhaler with these three oils and placed a bottle of Scots pine on a special place in Bea's room.

In the meantime, we had agreed that I would make a special composition for Bea, with oils that would on the one hand help her protect herself and on the other hand help her open herself up to her final journey.

Although I had said that I would send the composition by mail, Ina's story and the beautiful mail I received afterwards describing how Bea trusted me to choose the right oils made me decide to deliver it to her in person. I felt that I wanted to be near her. Perhaps because, at the end of her life, we could still mean something important to each other.

I found it a great honour that this wonderful wo-man could fine the energy to receive me. Sitting outside on the balcony I read to her which oils I had selected for her and why:

Spikenard – to bring comfort in deep sorrow, to intensify feelings of togetherness and acceptance, to protect during an abundance of stimuli and negative energy, ideal for use in people who are paranormal or highly intelligent;

Mountain lavender – to bring balance and peace and to protect against strong emotions and external impressions;

Sweet marjoram CO2 – in case of spiritual and emotional clinging, to help catch your breath and come to yourself, in the here and now and in the later;

Olibanum CO2 – to deepen breathing, bring rest, and establish a connection with the higher power;

Scots pine – purifying in case of negative thoughts and energies, to create air, space and peace;

Myrtle – for air and space on all levels, in case of tightness of body, mind and soul, to have spiritual oppression slip away;

Angelica seed CO2 – to bring balance together with the other oils and in order to be open to angelic energy;

Cypress – ideal for use during all transition processes;

Rose – for saying goodbye, bringing comfort, and establishing connection with the universal love that transcends everything, beyond all boundaries and limitations, in this life and beyond;

Neroli – to help during spiritual crises and when the skin has become thin on all levels;

Lemon balm CO2 – a powerful protector for highly sensitive people and a companion on the journey from this life to the next.

Saying goodbye, I wrote the following:

"Dear Bea,

These fragrant oils are meant to give you air and space, to help you find peace and come back to yourself, and to protect you while still being able to open yourself up to the transition from this life to the next. They will protect your energy field against excessive stimuli, without having you lock yourself within yourself. Breathe deeply – both in an emotional and in a spiritual sense. Wrap your-self in the fragrant coat of light and space, and know that you are safe. Have a good journey.

Love, Madeleine".

Through Ina, Bea let me know that she thought of our joint efforts as special and wonderful. Bea left a deep impression on me – and on everyone who remembers her with love. The ten minutes that I was allowed to share with her are among the most special moments of my life.

Thank you Bea.

This is one of my favourite, and relatively simple, blends for calmness and inner peace:

Spikenard (Indian) 15%, Marjoram sweet CO2 (Origanum majorana) 15%, olibanum CO2 (Boswellia carterii) 15%, lavender high alt 10%, rose distilled or CO2 (Rosa damascena) 10%, sandalwood (Indian) 10%, neroli 10%, mandarin 10%, bergamot 5%.

Also suitable for children from 1 year of age. Precautionary, avoid (spikenard) (application to the skin) during pregnancy and concomitant use of buspirone and antipsychotics such as haloperidol.

Case - Lea: aromacare and epilepsy

In recent years, I have gained good experiences with a combination of spikenard and other sedative oils, including clary, in epilepsy. Lea suffered from epilepsy due to brain damage at birth. Lea slept poorly and had many episodes during the night. The combination, including olibanum, clary and mandarin, gave her a much better quality of sleep, while she also had less nightly insults. It sufficed to use the inhaler before going to sleep. As a result, Lea was better able to rest and functioned better during the day.

Blend to assist (!) in the treatment for epilepsy:

Spikenard (Nardostachys jatamansi) 40%, Lemongrass (Cymbopogon flexuosus) 30%, Roman chamomile 10% (Anthemis nobilis), Sweet marjoram CO2 extract (Origanum majorana) 10%, Neroli(Citrus aurantium var. amara) 10%.

Note: *Suitable for suitable from 2 years of age. Precautionary, avoid (spikenard) during pregnancy and concomitant use of antipsychotics like haloperidol, lithium, and stimulants like methylphenidate.*

About Madeleine:

My name is Madeleine Kerkhof-Knapp Hayes. I am the founder and the chair of Kicozo, the Knowledge Institute for Complementary (Nursing) Care, here in The Netherlands. It is accredited by the Board of Nursing's Quality Registry. I am a member of several organisations, such as the Dutch Nurses Society, Palliactief and other bodies in palliative and dementia care, and the American Holistic Nurses Association.

Furthermore I am the chairperson of De Levensboom Foundation, a registered charity in palliative care, that supports patients in palliative stages in various ways. Palliative and terminal care have my special interest and expertise. I am passionate about the integration of complementary care in modern nurses (or other professional) care and mean stream healthcare.

I also own De Levensboom, Centre for Complementary Care (www.levensboom.com), where we provide clients such as nurses, hospitals nursing homes and hospices with high quality essential oils, CO2 extracts, base oils and a range of aromatic ready-made products.

Some thirty years ago I first started training to be a nurse. The main reason to leave the hospital was that I wanted to care for patients in a more holistic way, especially for the most fragile patients and the terminally ill. After I left nursing I gained a wealth of experience and expertise in natural orientated health care. I also trained and worked as a herbalist, hydrotherapist and aromatherapist. In 2003 I started training nurses and other health professionals on complementary nursing care techniques. I give one day workshops, as well as comprehensive three day courses and a full year training. I give talks and presentations. I also train non-professional carers in simple complementary techniques. Nowadays I mainly teach, both at my own school and on location throughout The Netherlands and abroad (English and/or German spoken). You can find more information on that on http://www.kicozo.nl/welcome/training-program/.

Therefore I published my book "Complementary Nursing in End of Life Care, Integrative Care in Palliative Care" in English in June 2015. You will find more information on the book and its availability in the EU and the rest of the world on http://www.kicozo.nl/welcome/the-book/.

Malte Hozzel

Malte and I are skype buddies! We have been trying to meet up in person for months, but something always gets in the way. The man jetsets across the planet like no-one else I know. Last time we spoke, he was in Columbia, he has written this from his training school in Provence.

He and I were introduced by Jonathan Hinde, who runs the UK division of Oshadhi. I had approached them to see if they would like to circulate my free book to their mailing list and we instantly became friends.

Both Malte and Jonathan come at aromatherapy from a similar angle to me, their backgrounds being in meditation studies. They like to understand the nature and spirituality of a plant, and to understand it vibrationally.

Malte has a unique slant on vibrational healing. Some of you may have seen his videos about the chemical constituent ketones and how they are dis-incarnators. It is fascinating stuff. Together, Oshadhi have amassed the most incredible selection of essential oils I have ever seen and boy, are they sublime. They tend to be from artisan producers, often are organic or wildcrafted and are always distilled very slowly to enable the largermoleculesto come through. I am biased, I like the UK site the best. If you cannot find what you are looking for on the US website, change .com to .co.uk and I promise you Jonathan will sort it for you. He promises the shipping won't be prohibitive! Sign up to their mailing list too. I can't tell you how muchI learn from their token mails to my inbox.

Spikenard by Dr Malte Hozzel

SPIKENARD with its Latin name *Nardostachys jatamansi* is native to the humid Himalaya regions and grows in the wild of Nepal, Bhutan, and Sikkim in mountain regions up to 3000-5000 m, other varieties are also found in China and Japan. The name « *jatamansi* »means « *bestower of life* » in Sanskrit and indicates how much this wonderful medicinal plant and its essential oil has been appreciated in the Ayurvedic ethnobotanical pharmacopeia of ancient India since ages. Being related to Valerian it belongs to the Valerianaceae plant family and resembles to some degree the Indian Valerian in fragrance and effect. Spikenard is a perennial herb with a strong wooden root and a long shoot of 10-60 cm.

The essential oil is obtained through steam distillation of the crushed and dried rhizome and roots of the herb. 100kg of the plant yields 1l of the essential oil. It is pale yellow in colour and medium in viscosity.

The main chemical ingredients are *bornylacetate, valeranone, jonon, tetramenthyloxatriccylodecanol,menthylthymyl-ether and 1,8-cineol*. The fragrance can be described as aromatic, earthy and spicy connected with a warm note. It blends well with Lavender, Lemon, Clary sage, Neroli, Patchouli and Vetiver.

In antiquity, maybe already since the epoche of Hammurabi (2000 BC), Spikenard was regarded as sacred and used for rituals as described in the Songs of Solomon, being reserved for kings and priests or initiates only. And in the New Testament we learn about the anointment of Jesus by Mary of Bethany before the Last Supper. It was an ancient custom to honour eminent guests by anointing their head and feet with Spikenard bearing witness of the high esteem the essential oil was held within those cultures. The fragrance was applied to relieve of fear and anxieties and preparing the body for burial. The value of the precious oil could be compared with the annual income of an average person at that time. Later it was also used as a valuable component in products for beauty care and in perfumes in connection with other flower scents by wealthy women in Ancient Egypt and Rome for example. The old trade routes made the essential oil available to the different countries of those days' world. Also today Spikenard is used for wound healing and skin care, mainly mature skin.

Experiences and research on Spikenardshow evidence of anti-inflammatory, antiseptic, antipyretic, calmative, sedative, laxative and tonic therapeutic properties. Essential oils consist of very small molecules granting healing powers to the deepest levels of our physical bodies and our consciousness as a whole. By virtue of their structural complexity and elaborated nature these substances with their volatile character are suited to fulfill manifold functions by just inhaling their fragrance or apply the essential oil to the skin. Modern medicine with their pharmaceutical chemical formula cannot compose the healing qualities essential oils unfold within the bodies of human beings. These treasures of Mother Nature carry the very being and essence of the original plant they are obtained from. They are light carriers blessed with the divine gifts of life force, intelligence and vibratory energies, characteristics which pharmaceutical products do not possess. Apart from that, essential oils do not load the body with undesirable side effects like so many conventional drugs do but rather convey manifold positive side effects.

The essential oil of Spikenard reveals antispasmodic effects in general, it has strong healing effects in case of epilepsy and is able to slow down the heart beat, strengthen the heart, compensate arrhythmia and regulate circulatory conditions meaning it has anti-hypertensive capabilities especially when combined with Ylang Ylang. It balances the hormonal system and helps with stomach disorders. Spikenard unfolds soothing qualities within the complete nervous system resembling those of Valerian. Therefore also those suffering from insomnia may receive relief. Furthermore all organs with the digestive tract included get balanced through the herb's activity and healing powers.

Logically, the conclusion follows that Spikenard is gifted with calming and soothing properties on the psychic level also. It is able to again stabilize the nervous system, also if hysterical conditions are the problem and to regenerate the mind after extreme exhaustion. It is a good choice in case inner steadfastness is required. Thus it is able to create interaction between the physical and the psychic side of our consciousness and may be helpful to reach deeper zones during meditation, too. The root aspect of the plant helps us to keep our feet anchored to the ground whereas the scent uplifts the soul to return to its divine source.

Dr.Malte Hozzel was born in Germany in 1944, and received his Ph.D. in 1979 from Heidelberg University in world literature and linguistics.

As a disciple of the famous Indian Master Maharishi Mahesh Yogi and as a teacher of Transcendental Meditation Dr. Hozzel has lectured on the TM programs in various European and overseas countries since 1972, established a number of TM-Centers and TM-Retreat-Academies in Germany, France and Belgium, and published several articles and books on the collective transformation of modern society. Malte and his wife spent several years with TM groups near Maharishi in several European Countries.

Over the years, Dr. Hozzel has had two particular fascinations: Research into the essential nature of plants with particular emphasis on aromatherapy and research into the effects of Yoga on consciousness. During this time his studies on aromatherapy became more and more a major focus of his interest. In 1990 he founded in Germany with his wife Véronique AYUS Essential Oils Intl. with the goal to create an int. market for high quality aromatherapy products and to expand his global contacts through lecturing on the effects of essential oils. Over the years AYUS' products have become one of the world's purest collection of essential oils, known to the experts for its wide range of rare specy essential oils and a large variety of other aromatherapy products which today comprise several brand names of essential oils lines distributed in 35 countries.

Dr. Hozzel's aromatherapy classes have been spreading systematically the knowledge of essential oils on an intl. level – and this mainly since 1995 thanks to his famous Aromatherapy Seminar Center situated on a property of 150 acres in the UNESCO protected area of Mont Ventoux in High Provence.

www.oshadhi-provence.com www.ortodeprouvenco.com

Fai Chan

If you thought I was productive with my time, you should meet my friend Delicia (her Chinese name is Fai). She is translating my books into Chinese and she is the voice of my conscience. If I think for even a second I am working hard I get a message off her and that soon puts me straight. She is a whirlwind of ideas and the networking queen having being able to secure herself a sponsorship from Gucci!

I swear she never sleeps. She lives in the US, networks and sells in China and chats to me in the UK. Love her, I do. And here's the thing, I would not dare be ill her presence she would shove me off the couch and get me back to work again! That being said, if it is worth knowing you can guarantee she has some aromatic knowledge about it.

Take a Step Backwards and Give Yourself a Break

Releasing Your Stuffed Emotions by Fai Chan

Without proper outlets, your stuffed emotion can turn to emotional issues such as anxiety, depression, bipolar disorder and so on. My client in this case study has long term bipolar disorder syndrome. Suffered by ups and downs in her life, she accumulated many unreleased emotions. This is further complicated by the fact that she did not like to do any exercise. Rarely can she find any outlets to let those unhealthy feelings out. Since she is a good cook, what she does for her pleasure is cooking and writing recipes. She also experiences heart palpitations from time to time. This makes her heart "weak" and "tight", as she termed it. She loves spicy food. That aggravates her symptoms.

The application of essential oils tends to be individually tailored as people have different preferences and protocols used. I am a very religious person. Since Spikenard and Frankincense were mentioned in the Bible, I pay special attention to them. I believe that those two, when properly combined with other essential oils, can make an effective blend to tackle her emotional issues.

To tackle her issues, the following blend is used:

- 2 drops Spikenard (*Nardostachys jatamansi*)
- 2 drops Frankincense (*Boswellia frereana*)
- 1 drop Helichrysum (*Helichrysum italicum*)
- 1 drop Roman Chamomile (*Chamaemelum nobile*)
- 1 oz (30ml) Jojoba oil

Spikenard: High in sesquiterpenes, this oil is very calming and anti inflammatory. It calms the CNS (Central Nervous

System), helps calm the mind, induces sleep, and brings the feeling of tranquility.

Frankincense: uplifting, revitalizing, centering, and anti-inflammatory. Since she has mood swings, she needs some invigorating oil. Frankincense is a healing oil. By adding it to the blend, it can enhance the healing of her past.

Helichrysum: Tonic to the body. It helps the client to tonify weaknesses in emotions and body. Renowned for wound healing, it can help heal the wound of the present and the past. It is emotionally balancing; it is able to stabilize the mood and to release any stuffed or suppressed emotions of the client.

Roman Chamomile: Calming and soothing to the CNS (Central Nervous System), Roman Chamomile can ease overthinking and hyperactivity. It is also a healing oil. This fact enables it to further calm the stress and tension of the client.

Application Method: 2-3 times a day by applying on the neck, and the chest.

After the first application, she found her heart palpitations disappeared, she felt so calm and soothing. She also slept well. Forgetting some applications did not make her situation worse. She kept applying at least twice a week, however.

She used to have tight shoulders. After using the blend, she felt relaxed and did not experience much muscle tension or pain.

Since she did not do any exercise, I suggested her to go to steam room to release her stuck energy. She listened to my suggestion, went to steam room twice a week. She told me that she felt so relieved after that.

She is still taking medications, but she has reduced them to the minimum dosage.

After two weeks using the blend, she becomes a happier and bright person.

It is worth mentioning that the look of her her skin has also improved although she has not applied the blend onto her face. It enhances her confidence.

Her positive energy seems to attract positive energy to her. It seems to her that her circumstances are getting better, she has more friends now. Perhaps, it is her change from inside out that makes her more courageous to face reality and future.

Spikenard brings warmth and endurance to her life. This improves her EQ (Emotional Quotient) in handling the harshness in her life. With her positive change in attitude, things become more enviable and amicable to her. God may not take away her hardship, but HE did send a helper, in this case the Spikenard blend, to help her see things in balance.

Fai Chan (CMAIA)

Fai Chan started her career in 2014, and currently, she has published 10 articles with international journals. She has recently published two books in Chinese in China, and is the publisher of the digital Chinese aromatherapy journal -- Aroma Search. A Chinese publisher is very interested in her work and would like her to write for it.

Recently, she has signed a contract to write a chapter in Jack Canfield's forthcoming book -- The Road To Success. He is the co-author of the Chicken Soup for the Soul series. She will be inducted into the National Academy of Best Selling Authors, and will attend the award ceremony in Hollywood in September.

The Wall Street Journal is arranging an interview with her. She will appear in the TV show(s) for an interview in Hollywood in the second half of the year.Since she started posting on weibo (the largest Chinese social media), her posts have regularly been hot picks.

She is a clinical member of the Alliance of International Aromatherapists. Serving in serves on the board of one of the world's leading aromatherapy association, she is the chair of the publication committee.

She is now translating the articles into Chinese for IJPHA (International Journal of Professional Holistic Aromatherapy) to enable then to presence in China, Hong Kong, and Taiwan.

Aiding leading aromatherapists to translate their work into Chinese she is helping them to promote their books as well as co-authoring with them.Some of her work can be found via Academic Search Engine EBSCOhost.

Her company Deli Aroma LLC is dedicated to holistic healing protocols. Her specialities are mainly in the healing of emotional issues with aromatherapy. Based on Traditional Chinese Medicine

(TCM) *framework, with the synergistic effects of combining the therapeutic approach with chemistry, her remedies are very effective. She takes joy in knowing her clients personally, and gives them personalized care. She dedicates a lot of time and effort in doing follow-ups, asking many questions and firmly she believes that, when they are healed, they will thank her for that.*

When people are sick, they may not know the best treatment. As a therapist, she is very clear what works best.

Email: deliaroma8@gmail.com

Profile: http://ezinearticles.com/expert/Fai_Chan/2259684

Alan Howell

I met Alan when I was lecturing in Beijing. We had just been to a dinner hosted by Danièlle Ryman and the lady who was my translator Ruonan Shi, and we had not yet been able to speak. We said hello as we left the restaurant, both of us feeling mildly embarrassed that we had ignored the other. Alan and his husband Alex had me absolutely in fits in the minibus home.

The next day they came to my rescue from a nervous day trapped in the hotel when I gatecrashed their trip to The Forbidden City. Even after spending a day with them both, fighting to get photos of thrones, riding in horse drawn carriages and climbing up to shrines, I had no understanding just how clever he was.

Then he took the stage after me on the last day of the conference. He arrived with his hair streaked bright blue and proceded to juggle as a means of showing how energy worked. His lecture about the energies of medicine was incredible...and delivered at the fastest speed you have ever seen. I fell instantly in love with both him and Alex! This grew even deeper when, after I had arrived home and they had stayed another day, I found they had bought tea made of rose buds from The Great Wall and sent them back to Ludlow for me.

Alan sells essential oils and also wonderful elemental blends. They are like something from another planet! I adore them. Please do visit his website (full of loads more information) and consider buying buy some of his blends. You will never see medicine in the same way.

Let's see what he has to say...

Spikenard with its musky deep aroma is lifted by the sweet rising energies of its lighter terpenes. There is no mistaking the underlying valerianol and nardol aromas that cause people to so often confuse this oil with Valerian, however these are in tiny proportions and Spikenard is so much more than this. With around 30% alpha-gurjunene with its distinctive wood balsam depth, and almost another 30% of patchoulene with its also distinctive balsamic earthy rich aroma, you would be forgiven for placing this oil firmly in Wood Element or at least leaning to Earth. It is only in re-visiting this oil and spending time with it, that it eventually opens up its higher qualities. As the base earthy notes become familiar, the olfactory system starts to detect the sweeter higher terpenes and tones of aging lemon are lifted by spicy notes of cardamum and ginger. It is these spicy notes that show the true Fire Element quality of Spikenard. I would consider Spikenard to have a primary action in Fire Element supported by a secondary action in Wood. It is these qualities that places Spikenard essential oil significantly apart from Valerian. With a primary action in Fire it should never be a substitute for Valerian which is most definitely a primarily Water Element oil. There is no doubting the Wood Element quality that they both share but it is this fundamental opposition in primary action that allows these oils to have very different actions and uses.

In conditions such as depression, which often result as an excess of Metal Element, Valerian is often prescribed. This will add to the Water Element and block the free-flow of energy in the creative cycle from Metal Element thus adding to the Metal excess and commonly resulting in a hangover style headache hours later which is a symptom of the Water excess.

Spikenard is an ideal choice for the Metallic individual who is in the depths of despair. The powerful Fire Element primary action of Spikenard melts the Metal, whilst the secondary action of Wood helps to further draw the Metal Element through the control cycle and thus assists the stimulation of energy flow.

This whole process facilitating a restoration to natural balance: It is in understanding the powerful Fire Element of Spikenard that we can see why it comes into its own in extreme depressive conditions such as manic depression, febrile delirium, delirium tremens, migraine, stress tension and bipolar depression.

It is interesting that jatamansone semi-carbazone, a sesquiterpene ketone isolated from the rhizome has been used in the treatment of various delirium states, and whilst there is a presence of jatamansone in the oil, it is the understanding of the energetic qualities that allows us to see how this oil best works in its whole state rather than in chemical isolation.

A deeper understanding of the Fire Element inspires a better comprehension of the processes of homoeostasis. In Chinese medicine the Fire Element governs the Triple Heater which in the West we understand as the body's homoeostatic principles. Now we can truly begin to see why Spikenard's Fire Element is so powerful in helping the body to stabilise and regulate. So many of the traditional therapeutic qualities of Spikenard are regulatory in nature, supporting: mood swings, bipolar depression, panic attacks, balancing Sympathetic nervous system and Parasympathetic nervous system functions, assisting regular heartbeat, arythmia, emotional regulator and helping to avoid menstrual disturbances.

The Fire Element also governs the Heart Constrictor which in the West we know as the pericardium. This is the protective area around the heart, and thus emotionally is imperative to keep us protected and to ensure a sense of emotional security.

In Chinese medicine the Heart Constrictor protects the heart from excessive emotional outbursts from the bodies seven emotions (anger, joy, grief, anxiety, pensiveness, fear and shock) and prevents damage and long-term paroxysms which can be the cause of disease.

Once again we can see how Spikenards' Fire Element helps us to maintain emotional and hence physical stability by supporting the functions of both Triple Heater (homoeostasis) and the Heart Constrictor (pericardium). Remembering that Chinese Medicine sees the Mind as being housed in the Heart, we can see why Spikenard is often used to support mind body interactions such as general stress and anxiety, insomnia, agitation and panic attacks.

An imbalance in the Metal Element can often be the cause of skin, nail and digestive problems, as the Lung (and skin) and Large Intestines are governed by the Metal Element. Since an excess of Metal Element can result in an over active skin organ, applying Spikenard with its melting Fire Element can often bring relief to such skin conditions as acne, eczema, scleroderma, hives and psoriasis. It has also been traditionally used for skin allergies and rejuvenating skin conditions, although these conditions tend not to be as a result of Metal excess, they can be due to lack of circulation to the peripheral blood vessels and hence Spikenards Fire qualities will help to stimulate peripheral blood flow and the complexion as a whole.

Spikenard has also been used historically to support healthy hair, and it is again its regulating relationship to the Metal Element that best supports this (since Metal Element is expressed externally by body hair). It is also said to help restore colour to grey hair, and since is the colour of excess

Metal, a melting of the Metal may indeed allow natural hair colour to be restored.

We must not forget Spikenards' secondary action of Wood Element, and although this is rarely exhibited in Spikenards therapeutic qualities it is always an underlying support as it too helps to draw excess Metal Element via the control cycle. It is in this Element that we can see the effects on the muscular system and how Spikenard is able to ease muscular aches and pains, support connective tissue problems and ease rheumatic conditions.

If an individual is lacking Wood Element and hence suffers any of the above conditions, Spikenard will not only provide a source of Wood Element, but in also providing more Fire Element too, the body will need less Wood Element to convert to Fire energy. This results in a supported stable supply of Wood Element with no disruption to the Fire Element. The overall effect of this will be to support the lacking muscular/connective tissue problems whilst helping to create a stable flow in the creative cycle and hence support a healthy eco-system that is the human body.

Spikenard would rarely be a first choice for these conditions, but in any individual suffering these minor symptoms alongside other emotional, regulatory disturbances Spikenard would come into its own.

It has a direct effect into both the Heart and Crown Chakras. The obvious connection between the Heart Chakra and Fire Element is clear from our understanding of the Heart Constrictor, but the Crown Chakra takes a little further explanation. The Crown Chakra is our doorway home, it is the point that we can use to see spiritually, it is closely connected to the pineal gland.

French philosopher Descartes described the pineal gland as the 'principle seat of the soul' and this fits closely with ancient understandings of the Chakras. It is known that the pineal gland responds to light stimulation and is consequently well named as the third eye, although popular understanding of the Chakras says that the Brow Chakra is the Third eye.

It is in actuality the connection between the Brow (forehead) Chakra and the Pituitary gland, in union with the Crown Chakra and the Pineal gland, that together allow the Third Eye to see. Responsive to light, the pineal gland is known to be the regulator of our daily and seasonal circadian rhythms along with our sleeping and waking patterns through the secretion of melatonin. This gland also governs the gonadotrophins and is responsible for the development and functioning of the ovaries and testes. Now we can see more clearly how Spikenard is related to both the Heart and Crown Chakras.

Spikenard is known to be beneficial to the regulation of the hormonal system and the stimulation of the ovaries, we have already looked at the number of regulatory functions Spikenard can support in the systems of; cardiovascular, lymphatics, emotional, genito-urinary and mind-body qualities.

Understanding the relationship of the pineal gland to the Crown Chakra helps us to comprehend how Spikenard is able to support the body's functions of balance as well as supporting homoeostasis through the Fire Element. This connection with the pineal gland and its function of melatonin secretion also shows how Spikenard is able to support rested sleep function and relinquish insomnia.

Each of the Chakras is divided into seven sub-chakras and when we look at the seventh (spiritual) sub-chakra of the Heart chakra we can see where Spikenard is most specific within the Chakra system. The Spiritual sub-chakra of the Heart Chakra is the point where we achieve spiritual enlightenment without thought process. The use of Spikenard during meditation practice can therefore assist in the meditative art of reaching spiritual enlightenment without thought process, and it may be this connection that has given this oil the tradition of inspiring devotion, creating deep inner peace and aiding spiritual learning.

In zoopharmacognosy Spikenard is a popular oil with cats who are no doubt attracted to the valerianal and nardol reminiscent to Valerian but it is the actinidine in both plant oils that make some cats excited or even slightly aggressive. Spikenard has similar effects in other mammals as it does in humans, and so its implications are much the same.

It is an oil always worth considering for self-selection wherever there is an indication of irregularities or rhythmic disturbances. It is also worth considering when there are very strong rhythmic behaviour patterns such as constant kicking or nuzzling, as correction and realignment to the circadian rhythms may help resolve this. Since Valerian is banned under FEI (Federation Equestre Internationale) it seems another good reason to consider Spikenard for self-selection when working with equines who appear to need sedation. I have known several horses select Spikenard when there is a history of malaise and depressive states. Spikenard is amazing at finding the root of emotional disturbances and supporting the lifting of the spirit to a point of balance and contentment.

Bibliography:

- A Handbook of Aromatic and Essential Oil Plants Cultivation, Chemistry, Processing and Uses; Bedi, Tanuja & Vyas
- A Handbook of Medicinal Plants A complete Sourcebook; Prajapati, Purohit, Sharma & Kumar
- Aromatherapy Book, The; Jeanne Rose
- Aromatherapy Practitioner Reference Manual, The; Sylla Sheppard-Hanger
- How Animals Heal Themselves; Caroline Ingraham

Alan Howell studied Herbal Medicine in 1985, interested in the energetics of plant material he redirected his study towards subtle energy medicine.

Alan studied at the British School of Shiatsu- Do and qualified as a Shiatsu practitioner. His desire to work holistically means that his bodywork is now augmented by nutritional and environmental advice. This combination of Herbal, Nutritional, Environmental and Bodywork is all driven by a desire to harmonise the body's energetic system. He specialises in a branch of Shiatsu known as Shin- Tai. Directly translated this means source- body, supporting optimum Physical, Emotional and Spiritual harmony.

Whilst studying Herbal Medicine, Alan was using essential oils internally. Unhappy with the quality of oils available on the retail market he started sourcing them himself. Alan now supplies an

336

extensive range of high quality oils to Professional Therapists. His work with subtle energy is reflected in the choice of Essential Oils, and is a priority in the storage and bottling process. For several years he supplied friends and colleagues with oils to use in their own practices, sharing costs and keeping prices low. The business grew by word of mouth and has resulted in a business in its own right. The philosophy has stayed the same though: to provide superior quality oils for therapists to use in their practice, with consideration to the end user (the client), and with care for the environment that is our home - Mother Earth.

All of the oils supplied are true to species and country of origin as printed on the label. Alan runs regular workshops on the Energetics of Essential Oils and their application to both humans and animals. http://www.shechina.co.uk/

Part 8 Recipes

The majesty of aromatherapy is never going to be found in someone else's recipe. Inflammation in the body comes from dis-ease of the spirit. The body cannot sleep because emotional and physical pains disturb the body. A good blend will be designed for the individual based on intuition, knowledge and a great deal of listening and compassion.

The magic of a blend too, has as much to do with the energy of its creator. Whether that is the soil it came from of the person who blended it. My same palliative blend would be lovely, but it would not carry the energy of Madeleine. Whether my patient would suffer for that remains to be seen, doubtless my spirit has something different to offer. I suspect the healing would not be less, only different.

A possible bi-product of this section might be your recognition of similar oils cropping up over and over again. This is a useful pattern to see. Spikenard may be in your cupboard now, but given its ecological crisis, while we want to keep buying for the sake of the Nepalese economy, it is useful to discover other medicines which might serve us just as well. After all, not every day offers saturnic lessons, thank

Goddess, perhaps we should conserve our bottle for those arduous days that do.

That said, if ancient wisdom is to be believed then the elixir in this particular bottle has a shelf life of three years. It would be a shame if we never got to use it up!

I am not going to teach you how to use essential oils here. If this is your first foray into aromatic lands, welcome. I hope you are enjoy your journey and will stay a while. Lessons on how to use your tools can be found in my free book The Complete Guide. Please take this opportunity to download it and learn from comprehensive instructions there.

These recipes, then, are simply my thoughts about how spikenard *could* be used. Learn them. Change them. Develop them. Become a better aromatherapist than I, because this section is merely a stepping stone to your own individual way of healing.

The contraindications are minimal here. I would advise avoiding spikenard, like all oils, during the first 16 weeks of pregnancy.

Sleep

4oz St John's Wort Carrier Oil

Spikenard x 2

Spearmint x 1

Valerian x
Rub into the neck and shoulders an hour before bed time.

Anxiety Blend

4oz blank lotion

Spikenard x 3

Camomile x 2

Neroli x 1

Rub into the inside of the wrist, where there is good blood supply and onto the neck three or four times daily. This blend also works beautifully in an aromapendant to wear around the neck throughout the day.

Shock

Spikenard x 1

Holy Basil x 1

Vetiver x 1

A drop of each in a warm bath. Soak for at least 20 minutes.

Inflammation

4oz (100ml) blank lotion

Spikenard x 2

Roman Camomile x 4

Basil Linalol x 1

Smooth gently into the affected area five times a day.

Pain

Spikenard x 1

Lavender x 4

Yarrow x 1

Smooth gently, into the affected area five times a day.

Perception of Pain

If the thought of pain is overwhelming, often it can make the *actual* pain worse too, so inhalations are useful to calm the mind and bring inflammatory markers down.

Diffuse:

Rose x 1

Spikenard x 1

Myrrh x 1

Antispasmodic

3oz Tamanu Carrier oil

1oz Sea Buckthorn Carrier Oil

Spikenard x 2

Clary Sage x 1

Lavender x 2

Emotional Stability

Spikenard x 2

Frankincense x 1

Lemon x 3

I like this one infusing in the living room!

Steadfast Will

4oz Blank Body Lotion

Spikenard x 1

Basil x 1

Sweet Orange x 2

I have been using this in a morning, as an all over after I have a shower. I designed it as a means of staying true to my New Year's Resolutions. We are in March, they are not broken and I have lost two stone! Also...my skin is very, very soft!

Epilepsy

Rose Absolute x 3

Spikenard x 1

Vetiver x 2

Use in a diffuser or blend into 4oz of grapeseed oil and massage into the shoulders and neck, morning and evening.

Contraindications: Omit rose during pregnancy

Flatulence

4oz Borage Carrier Oil

Spikenard x 1

Dill x 1

Carrot x 2

Massage into the abdomen, drawing a square around the navel with your fingers: two strokes up the left side, two, above the navel, two down the right, and one across the pelvis to follow the flow of food through the intestine. Use after meals or when the air becomes a little ripe!

Hypercholesterol

1oz Borage Carrier Oil.

Spikenard x 1

Rose Otto x 1

Rosemary x 2

Rub into the chest and wrists three times daily.

Contraindications: Omit rose during pregnancy

Palpitations

1oz Rosehip Carrier Oil

Rose Otto x 1

Spikenard x 1

Vetiver x 1

Contraindications: Omit rose during pregnancy

Jaundice

Not sure why I could not decide between the hepatic oils here, but I kept coming back with OR so, in the spirit of always listening to your intuition...

1 fl oz Borage Carrier

Spikenard x 1

Rosemary x 1

Carrot / Eucalyptus x 1

Respiratory

I am probably being a bit naughty here, since agarwood is a protected species. I was given a gift of some that been gained from sustainable resources of inoculated trees and the oil is utterly magical. It seems to have entirely healed my lungs. If you would like me to give you details of where you can get it, please feel free to drop me a line.

1 fl oz Evening Primrose Carrier Oil

Spikenard x 2

Agarwood (Aloes wood in the Bible) x 1

Frankincense x 2

Tension Headache

1 fl oz Pumpkin Seed Oil

Spikenard x 1

Vetiver x 1

Lavender x 1

This is a bit like using a sledgehammer to crack a nut but should the mood take you...

Rub into the neck and shoulders, as well as the temples and forehead during an attack.

ADHD

Vetiver x 2

Spikenard x 1

German Chamomile x 2

I would be inclined to get the Christmas Gifts book out and think of every possible way to use these oils. We could paint them onto unvarnished pencils for school, use them in a diffuser, have them on the child's drinks coaster. I think a steady ongoing exposure works better than the 30 min on / 30 min off diffusion protocol. Certainly...in the bath might mean they finally go to sleep and give you some respite!

Febrile Delirium

1 fl oz Spikenard Hydrolat

Mandarin x 1

Monarda x 1

Blissful Native American medicine, soak a face cloth, dab over the body to cool and soothe

Hypertensive

Spikenard x 1

Ylang Ylang x 1

Clary Sage x 1

Use in an aromapendant around the neck, or on an aromapatch to have ongoing exposure and reduce blood pressure.

Incidentally, for those of you who do not follow me on Facebook, my bp has come down from a terrifying 139/79 to 114/76 using clary sage and ylang ylang. Spikenard can only help to lower it more.

Fierce Menstrual Flow

Spikenard x 3

Rose x 1

Clary Sage x 2

This follows on from the advice in the rose and clary sage books, but here, spikenard would be indicated if the flow is very heavy and fast. That would indicate an excess of rhakta dhatu.

Winter Warmer

Dex and I have a daily ritual. He tells me he is too ill to go to school and I try to decide if he is lying! Most of the time, it is somewhere between the two. He has "winterfulness", he is cold and wants to stay under the covers. This is a lovely way to add a warm day to grey days, for no other reason than just because...!

1 fl oz blank lotion

Spikenard x 1

Ginger x 1

Cardamom x 2

Use any time, anywhere. Consider it a security blanket!

Summer Coolers

Conversely we can use spikenard to give us relief in the sun.

1 fl oz Rosewater

Spikenard x 1

Palmarosa x 1

Rose x 1

Splash it all over...gently, of course. These are treasures!

Contraindications: Omit the rose during pregnancy

Urge Incontinence

1 fl oz St John's Wort Carrier Oil

Spikenard x 1

Cypress x 1

Rose x 1

Massage into the abdomen and lower back, each time after visiting the toilet, to get a really good build up of oils.

Contraindications: No suitable for use during pregnancy

Somatic Disease

I run the risk of looking like I think all of these are only in the mind, by categorising these together. I don't. I do however think that they have their roots in emotional disease which are propagated by changes in neurotransmitters affecting inflammatory markers. In other words that stress makes them worse. As such then, these emotional diseases, I feel, work by very similar mechanisms.

Chronic Fatigue & ME

1 fl oz Black Seed Oil

Spikenard x 1

Helichrysm x 1

Bergamot x 1

Use for fully body massage, weekly to invigorate the system. Alternatively use as a daily massage oil on painful and weak areas.

IBS

1 fl oz Moringa Oil (the Ben Oil you see in the ancient recipes)

Spikenard x 1

Roman Camomile x 3

Cardamom x 1

Lemon x 1

90% of the body's serotonin is found in the gut. Since lemon oil influenced levels of this, modulating mood, this is designed to prevent your tum from being glum and to settle the digestion.

Use as an abdominal massage. Apply three times a day, drawing a square around the navel with your fingers: two strokes up the left side, two, above the navel, two down the right, and one across the pelvis to follow the flow of food through the intestine.

Fibromyalgia

Spikenard x 2

Helichrysm x 1

Basil linalool x 1

Smooth gently into the pain affected areas five times a day.

Skin care

For ease, all of these are in 4oz of moisturiser

Mature Skin

Spikenard x 1

Galbanum x 1

Neroli x 2

Greasy Skin

Spikenard x 1

Vetiver x 1

Petitgrain x 3

Poor skin after illness

Spikenard x 2

Helichrysm x 1

Rose x 2

Contraindications: Omit rose during pregnancy

Memory

1 fl oz Blank Lotion

Vetiver x 1

Rose x 3

Spikenard x 1

Rub into the neck three times a day, or onto the wrists if the neck is difficult. This blend would be good on a facecloth to inhale too.

Contraindications: Omit rose during pregnancy

Learning

Spikenard x 1

Bergamot x 3

Vetiver x 1

Use in a diffuser whilst studying. You will find the actual process of sitting and calculating becomes easier too, rather than speeding to get away from the homework.

Parkinson's Disease

We are aiming to reduce the symptoms here and to make the patient more comfortable.

1 fl oz Tamanu Carrier Oil

Spikenard x 6

Geranium x 3

Camomile Roman x 3

A beautiful massage to calm the spirit and reduce the tremors.

Sadness

Spikenard x 2

Melissa x 1

Rose Otto x 1

However you think, bath diffuser, massage oil, whatever you think you can get your patient to agree to.

Contraindications: Omit rose during pregnancy

Hair care

Spikenard x 2

Cedarwood x 1

Rosemary x 1

Add into 4fl oz shampoo, conditioner or massage oil.

Contraindications: Substitute lavender for rosemary in cases of high blood pressure.

Conclusion

Many of you will recall my blog post From www.thesecrethealer.com from March 9th 2015

March 2016

I did not forget, dear reader. What a journey I have had exploring this plant and its medicine. Not least because it has taken me so very long! The spikenard has helped though, because my patience and willpower has been fantastic. I hope never to find a book as hard to write as this one, and yet I also

I wish to always be as engaged and fascinated by the twists and turns it has taken.

When Christmas came I wrote about spikenard being the oil of anointment and it was like someone emptied a rubbish bin of ancient knowledge on my desk and declared "Here sort that lot out – because what you have written doesn't look right to me!"

It rankled me. The entire internet had spikenard pegged as the oil used, they even allegedly had Tutankhamen's tomb findings to substantiate the claims.

But you know that feeling you have when you can't quite put your finger on it but....

Certainly, it was not as cut and dried as it would seem. I could not get the information to stack up in my mind. Finally after hundreds hours of study, write, rewrite I can't imagine there isn't a stone that I haven't overturned. Hell, Dex and I have invented a new word for it. Unwrite – when they add it the lexicon it will have the definition "That moment when you realise three chapters are wrong because of a new piece of research that no-one has noticed before". It was unwritten no less than eight times! I am...eventually...happy.

Was it spikenard in the jar then?

Ah well, that's for the reader to decide surely?

Personally, I feel sure it was now, yes.

I couldn't help but wonder at how amazing its effects had been on me when I had used it 12 months ago. It made me think about this question we explored earlier as to why is it a plant might be able to heal a human. My own thoughts strayed to that stationary plant, on the mountainside, under the snow fighting for its very existence. Nearly extinct, it can do nothing but rely on the angels, its pollination so slow and sporadic. Somehow the species' recovery even seems saturnic, long, slow and very, very cold in that snow.

And day to day, it cannot run from the challenges it faces from yaks and illegal collectors, it remains locked still, with its roots firmly in one place and it has to face the world, despite at the threats that it faces. I couldn't help but smile at the synchronicity of how these metabolites help it to survive in a world where the environment is acting upon *it*. The wind rocks it, the snow buries it and any number of flying creatures, land, feed and they reproduce upon it. It seems to me this idea of things happening to the plant is very much the same as how stress attacks us on an everyday basis. It is our environment outside of our internal control. Nevertheless plants have evolved ways to co-exist in a symbiotic relationship with other species (whether that is plant life, insects or birds for example) in a peaceful symbiotic way. I have to hope that someday, we as a species can learn that too.

The book is dedicated to a remarkable family, Marlys, and her grandchildren Anthony, Joshua and Kayla who have found just such a symbiotic way. Family troubles hit Marlys in the most tragic way and suddenly she found herself looking after both of her daughter's children. Throughout the book I was aware of a connection I was making with her story; how she had stepped into the breach and just got on with things. Marlys is very special to me. She initially contacted me after reading one of my books, at the end of her tether because the boys were not sleeping. Vetiver soon put them straight!

My connection with her feels all the stronger because my work requires me to spend long periods of time alone. To hear a friendly voice in the wilderness helps a great deal. To all of you who send me messages through the months, I want to thank you too. They are a connection to the outside world on days when I am far too up in my head! They are appreciated and treasured.

I also want to thank my wonderful colleagues and associates for all the help they have given me with this one: Dr Malte Hozzel, Madeleine Knapp Hayes, Delicia Chan, Kelly Holland

Azzarro, Gergely Hollódi and Alan Howell who have so generously shared their knowledge and expertise. To Dr Lise Manniche for her wisdom about King Tut and for the pointer to Galen's kyphi recipe. I am indebted to you for always answering my questions and discretely ignoring my obvious envy for your job as an Egyptologist!

Lastly I want to thank Chris and Jeanne for their lovely gifts to me at Christmas, but particularly for Jeanne's beautiful pashmina. The second I held the purple and gold cloth in my hands the Phoenix seemed to soar into life. I have been wearing it everywhere with my royal blue coat. One night, the wind was so bitter when I was walking the dog, that I wrapped it around my head like Muslim girls wear theirs. Suddenly, I felt the cold nights of the Hebrews on their exodus, protected by the warmth of the silk. The scarf had been delayed for several weeks because she kindly re-ordered it for me, because the first was lost in the post. Had it come at the correct time, the symbolism would have been completely lost on me

Such strange co-incidences have raised themselves whilst I have been writing this book, but I'd like to share two of them with you. The first I shared with you on January 1st as a recipe, spikenard, basil and sweet orange for will power. Little did I know that because of those three oils by the tie I released this book, I would be two stone lighter. After a lifetime of struggling with my weight my cast iron will is shedding it like dead skin! Watch this space...

The second was in a time where I was considering themes of oppression and imprisonment, I was presented with a box of the most incredible treasures; a shoebox full of letters belonging to my grandparents when my grandfather was taken prisoner of war in Arnhem in the Second World War. There are literally hundreds of them and I never even know they existed. (And no, I didn't even know about them when I wrote about the woman and her incarcerated husband, so how weird is that?) My family have asked me to try and make a book out of them so I shall be away for a short while, whilst I continue to study a different dimension to the lesson I never even knew existed. Alongside that, I have just closed a deal with a company to offer online training courses. That paired with the fact I shall have to make videos of myself fills me with excitement and dread.

Meanwhile please do use the oil and send me your thoughts about the book. My favourite parts were the insect chemistry, the cholera epidemic and also finding out that David Don and Joseph Banks are now remembered on a stone plaque at 32

Soho Square, the former site of the Royal Society after all the contributions to botany. Please remember to post a review on Amazon or rave/ moan about it on social media, and tell us what your favourite part was too. The feedback really helps me to sell more books and to know how to write any future ones for you. Whilst these books are really only my studies into a plant, I hope that I always include what you want to read.

For now, I don't think I can be more eloquent than Celine and André and I'll ask them to sum up spikenard for us.

The   Prayer: https://www.youtube.com/watch?v=iJkq-U7_8ZA

Thanks so much again, and as ever don't forget to review and buy!

Bye

Liz xx

Picture overleaf:

Illustration of *Nardostachys grandiflora*

Joseph Dalton Hooker (1817-1911) - Curtis's botanical
magazine vol. 107 ser. 3 nr. 37 tabl. 6564 from
www.botanicus.org

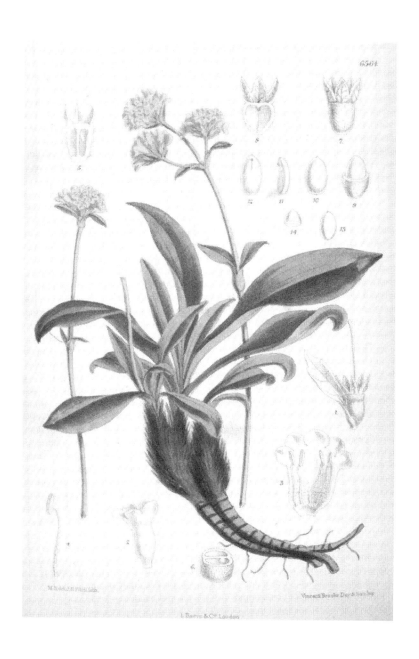

About the Author

Elizabeth Ashley is an international speaker for the International Federation of Aromatherapists and the UK Director for the National Association of Holistic Aromatherapists. She is a prolific writer of professional articles, in particular for the IFA magazine Aromatherapy Thymes, Aromatika.hu, NAHA Journal and Holistic Therapist She qualified as an aromatherapist in 1993, and then passed her Advanced Aromatherapy Diploma in 1994. She has been practicing aromatherapy for almost 25 years.

In 1999, she fell into a whole new career in the aggressive commercial sector of recruitment consultancy. There she discovered her father's second hand car salesman genes had passed along and found she had quite a gift of the gab! More than that, she discovered she could sell...and then some.

In 2008, Elizabeth fell ill during pregnancy with a blood clot in her lungs. The pulmonary embolism prevented her from working and she started to write. Very quickly she gained her first contract as a ghost writer...a recipe book for cheese cakes!

In 2010 she was published professionally for her work on Galbanum - (Ferula Galbaniflua) oil in the Aromatherapy Thymes, journal of the International Federation of

Aromatherapists, and on TubeRose - (Rosa damascena) oil by the New Zealand Register of Holistic Therapist.

In 2011 she was seconded on a consultative basis to Walsall Independent Treatment Centre, designed to be a rainbow bridge between traditional and complementary medicines. There she became aware of the rumblings of change in healthcare. Her book Sales Strategies for Gentle Souls explains the connotations of this.

Many of her books are aimed at helping qualified aromatherapists to expand their healing repertoire and build their businesses. She also writes for people who have an interest in essential oils and want to learn how to heal. Her in depth essential oil profiles chart the healing properties of plants from the most arcane depths of historic folklore up to the scientific lab trials of today.

She lives in Shropshire with her husband and youngest son, kept company by their Staffordhire Bull Terrier, Bella, the budgie and many shoals of tropical fish! Her elder son and daughter attend University and make her prouder than anything ever could. Elizabeth Ashley is The Secret Healer.

☐

Other Books by the Author

Why not check out my reviews?

75 Quick and Easy Aromatherapy Christmas Gifts Ideas: Essential Oil Recipes For Handmade Personalised Gifts

50 Easy Essential Oil Recipes for Skin Care Products for Dry Skin - Make Your Own Anti-Aging Moisturizers & Night Creams Professional Aromatherapy Skin Care Tips and Beauty Secrets

The Secret Healer Oils Profiles:

Some of the oils we have covered in this book will be familiar, but possibly not all. You may find some of the oils profiles deepen your knowledge and fascination for the art of aromatherapy.

Vetiver - (Vetiveria zizanoides): the Oil of Tranquillity

Monarda: A Native American Medicine

Holy Basil: An Ayurvedic Medicine

Rose - (Rosa damascena): Goddess Medicine; A Timeless Elixir

Sweet Basil - (Ocimum basilicum)– The Oil of Empowerment

Clary Sage- Salvia sclarea; Natural Estrogen?: Alleviate Symptoms of Menopause, Premenstrual Syndrome and Period Pains. Reduce Muscle Cramps And Restless Leg Syndrome. Ease Depression Symptoms and Improve Memory and Cognition with Clary Sage

The Secret Healing Manuals:

Book 1 - The Complete Guide to

Clinical Aromatherapy & Essential Oils for the Physical Body

Download for FREE

Book 2 Essential Oils for Mind Body Spirit

The Holistic Medicine of Clinical Aromatherapy

Book 3 The Essential Oil Liver Cleanse

The Professional Aromatherapist's Liver Detox

Book 4 The Professional Stress Solution

Essential Oils and Holistic Health Stress Management Techniques for The Professional Aromatherapist

Book 5 The Aromatherapy Eczema Treatment

Healing Eczema, Itchy Skin Rashes and Atopic Dermatitis with Essential Oils and Holistic Medicine

Book 6 The Aromatherapy Bronchitis Treatment

Support the Respiratory System with Essential Oils and Holistic Medicine for COPD, Emphysema, Acute and Chronic Bronchitis Symptoms

Sales Strategies for Gentle Souls; Targeted Sales Training for Professional Aromatherapists

Disclaimer

by SEQ Legal

(1)   Introduction

This disclaimer governs the use of this book. [By using this book, you accept this disclaimer in full. / We will ask you to agree to this disclaimer before you can access the book.]

(2)   Credit

This disclaimer was created using an SEQ Legal template.

(3)   No advice

The book contains information about aromatherapy and the use of essential oils.The information is not advice, and should not be treated as such.

[You must not rely on the information in the book as an alternative to qualified medical advice from a health professional. advice from an appropriately qualified professional. If you have any specific questions about any medical matter you should consult an appropriately qualified professional.]

[If you think you may be suffering from any medical condition you should seek immediate medical attention. You should never delay seeking medical advice, disregard medical advice, or discontinue medical treatment because of information in the book.]

(4)   No representations or warranties

To the maximum extent permitted by applicable law and subject to section 6 below, we exclude all representations, warranties, undertakings and guarantees relating to the book.

Without prejudice to the generality of the foregoing paragraph, we do not represent, warrant, undertake or guarantee:

that the information in the book is correct, accurate, complete or non-misleading;

that the use of the guidance in the book will lead to any particular outcome or result; or in particular, that by using the guidance in the book you will heal disease or work in any way as a cure for illness.

(5)   Limitations and exclusions of liability

The limitations and exclusions of liability set out in this section and elsewhere in this disclaimer: are subject to section 6 below; and govern all liabilities arising under the disclaimer or in relation to the book, including liabilities arising in contract, in tort (including negligence) and for breach of statutory duty.

We will not be liable to you in respect of any losses arising out of any event or events beyond our reasonable control.

We will not be liable to you in respect of any business losses, including without limitation loss of or damage to profits, income, revenue, use, production, anticipated savings, business, contracts, commercial opportunities or goodwill.

We will not be liable to you in respect of any loss or corruption of any data, database or software.

We will not be liable to you in respect of any special, indirect or consequential loss or damage.

(6)   Exceptions

Nothing in this disclaimer shall: limit or exclude our liability for death or personal injury resulting from negligence; limit or exclude our liability for fraud or fraudulent misrepresentation; limit any of our liabilities in any way that is not permitted under applicable law; or exclude any of our liabilities that may not be excluded under applicable law.

(7)   Severability

If a section of this disclaimer is determined by any court or other competent authority to be unlawful and/or unenforceable, the other sections of this disclaimer continue in effect.

If any unlawful and/or unenforceable section would be lawful or enforceable if part of it were deleted, that part will be deemed to be deleted, and the rest of the section will continue in effect.

(8)   Law and jurisdiction

This disclaimer will be governed by and construed in accordance with English law, and any disputes relating to this disclaimer will be subject to the exclusive jurisdiction of the courts of England and Wales.

(9)   Our details

In this disclaimer, "we" means (and "us" and "our" refer to) [Build Your Own Reality)] of [Sy8 1LQ].

A Very Brief Introduction to Ayurveda

This is just added in for people who needed a catch up earlier in the book.

Ayurveda is one of the most ancient medicine systems we have. It uses foods and meditations to cleanse and soothe the mind and body. It is a highly complex system of healing and although it is not my domain, it crosses into aromatherapy a great deal and can be very useful in understanding why people have a certain propensity to particular symptoms and disorders.

At the very dawn of our creation we develop our prakruti. It is believed this comes to us at conception and it remains with us throughout our lives. It never changes. We might refer to this is as the inherent character of a person, or perhaps their spirit.

Energy in the universe is separated into five different states in Ayurveda, and one or a combination of these can be applied to everything in existence.

- Earth

- Air

- Fire

- Water

- Ether

Our bodies and personalities also fall under this rule and it is classified and categorised into the three doshas, *vata*, *pitta*, *kapha*. Each of the bodily systems and also our personalities can be classified as such. In perfect health then there is a state of nothingness; that is there is *no excess* of any vata, pitta or kapha. The focus of Ayurveda is working with the body to try to reduce any excesses back into a state of nothingness or we might more easily understand this as balance. These ebb and flows within the body's energy are called the vikruti. Unlike pakruti, vikruti changes continually all through your life.

Vata

Is the connection between air and ether. It governs movement. It oversees the nervous system and the elimination systems of the body.

Words which describe vata are:

Light, cold, dry, rough, changeable, moving, quick

The vata physical frame is thin, light and slender. Their energy is quick and comes in very short burst. They can be prone to fatigue. They will feel the cold severely and their connective tissue, their skin, hair and teeth are dry and brittle. Their sleep is very light and the digestion is changeable.

When vata is unbalanced there is often weight loss, trouble sleeping, irritability, and joint problems such as arthritis.

Emotionally, vatas love new experiences and they bore very easily. Their tempers ignite very quickly, but also forgive at the same speed. When their energy is in balance they are wonderfully creative, happy to take initiatives in new ideas. They are eloquent conversationalists and are deliciously flexible people to be around; they are happy to go with the flow. What you will find though, is they are thinkers rather than doers and tend to be more interested in theories rather than practical applications of things.

When out of balance though vata energy makes worriers and these people in particular can really suffer from insomnia.

Pitta

Pitta controls digestion, metabolism and energy production. You can consider the primary function of this dosha to be that of transformation.

Words to describe pitta:

Hot, oily, fiery, sharp, inflamed, intense, penetrating, pungent

Physically Pittas are usually of fairly average size and weight. Many have bright red hair (remind you of anyone?), but you will often see their hair as thinning or balding too. They have the constitutions of an ox so they will believe they can eat anything and everything in the house. They have massive appetites and good enough digestion to deal with that. Their body temperature is warm. They have lustrous complexions with an almost oily sheen to it. Problems start when their pitta energy goes out of balance and they will suffer from sensitive skins and rashes. Their internal and external heat goes out of control leading to hot inflamed skins, burning cystitis or hot flushes. The first sign of the pitta imbalance will come when their digestion decides it has had enough and they start complaining of heartburn, and indigestion.

Pittas are very sharp witted and often can be a tad too outspoken and direct in their opinions. Because they are extremely concise they make excellent teachers and public speakers. They can concentrate very well and have very powerful intellects which make them clear, astute decision makers.

On a bad day they are short tempered and extremely argumentative.

Kapha

The primary function of kapha is protection and it governs the connective tissues of the body, the bones, muscles, fat and sinews

Words to describe kapha are:

Heavy, slow, soft, oily, steady, solid

Kapha are the big guys and gals. They have big builds and huge amounts of stamina. They have lovely soft eyes and almost oily sheens to their skins. They have thick and lustrous hair.

Emotionally they are steady people, completely reliable and very calm. They are thoughtful and loving and they are most comfortable with a steady routine. Emotional imbalance of kapha though will lead to stubbornness and burying their heads in the sand. Of all the doshas this one is the most resistant to change with these people staying in jobs and relationships long after they have outgrown them.

When kapha is in balance they are good sleepers and have excellent digestion but when kapha builds, the digestion becomes more sluggish and the sleep seems to go on and on.

They simply get slower and slower and harder to move! Often these people can suffer from diabetes, asthma and depression.

Just as the wind can move the earth, as sand across the desert, and ripples across the water, so vata controls and dominates the other doshas.

Most important for you to know is that vetiver pacifies vata and it reduces pitta.

In the West we find it very easy to become enthralled by plants with beautiful showy flowers, but the roots are not so exciting. In Ayurveda though, the root is recognised as the place where goodness of the plant is most concentrated. It's probably the plant part that provides the largest number of their medicines.

They are also used extensively in cooking and are ground to make medicinal powders.

Works Cited

1. (n.d.). Retrieved 03 01, 2016, from McClintock Bible Dictionary: https://bible.prayerrequest.com/7914-mcclintock-john-strong-james-cyclopedia/44720/

2. Adams, F. (1844). *The Seven Books of Paulus Aegineta: Translated from the Greek.* Sydenham Society.

3. Alexander von Humboldt, C. J. (1821). *An Illustration of the Genus Cinchona.* J. Searle ... and Longman, Hurst, Rees, Orme, and Brown.

4. Alleyne, J. (1733). *A New English Dispensary In Four Parts.* T. Astley & S. Austen,.

5. al-Tilmīd, H. A. (2007). *Aqrābādīn.* BRILL.

6. Alwis, A. P. (2011). *Celibate Marriages in Late Antique and Byzantine Hagiography.* A&C Black.

7. Amritpal Singh, A. K. (2009). *Nardostachys Jatamansi DC. Potential Herb with CNS Effects.* Retrieved 03 02, 2016, from Informatics Journals: http://www.informaticsjournals.org/index.php/ajprhc/article/view/633

8. Anderson, M. (2010). *Diary of Ancient Rites, A Guide For The Serious Practitioner.* CreateSpace Independent Publishing Platform.

9. Anupama. (2015, 10 15). *Medicinal uses of Nardostachys Jatamansi.* Retrieved 03 01, 2016, from bimbima: http://www.bimbima.com/health/post/2014/10/15/medicinal-uses-of-nardostachys-jatamansi.aspx

10. Arnold, E. A. (2009). *As Long as Space Endures: Essays on the Kalacakra Tantra in Honor of H. H the Dalai Lama.* Snow Lion Publications.

11. Askinson, G. W. (2003). *Perfumes and Their Preparation.* Wexford College Press.

12. Astma, A. J. (n.d.). *Phoinix.* Retrieved 02 11, 2016, from Theoi:

    http://www.theoi.com/Thaumasios/Phoinix.html

13. Authors: Subashini, R., Ragavendran, B., Gnanapragasam, A., Kumar Yogeeta, S., & Devaki, T. (2007). *Biochemical study on the protective potential of Nardostachys jatamansi extract on lipid profile and lipid metabolizing enzymes in doxorubicin intoxicated rats.* Retrieved 03 02, 2016, from Ingenta Connect:

http://www.ingentaconnect.com/content/govi/phar
maz/2007/00000062/00000005/art00013

14. *Bennu.* (n.d.). Retrieved 02 11, 2016, from Phoenix
Arises:
http://www.Phoenixarises.com/Phoenix/legends/be
nnu.htm

15. Bhishma P. Subedi, P. L. (2014). *Private Sector
Involvement and Investment in Nepal's Forestry Sector.*
Multi Stakeholder Forestry Programme.

16. Biren Shah, A. S. (2012). *Textbook of Pharmacognosy and
Phytochemistry.* Elsevier Health Sciences.

17. Black Phoenix Alchemy Lab. (n.d.). *Spikenard* .
Retrieved 02 11, 2016, from
http://blackPhoenixalchemylab.com/product-
tag/spikenard/

18. Blane, G. (1790). *Account of Nardus Indica or Spikenard.*
London: Royal Society.

19. Blane, G. (1790). Account of The Nardus Indica.
Philosophical Transactions of the Royal Society of London ,
pp. Vol. 80 (1790), pp. 284-292.

20. Blank, D. R. (2011). *The Experience of Jewish Liturgy: Studies Dedicated to Menahem Schmelzer*. BRILL.

21. Bloomfield, M. (1990). *Hymns of the Atharva-Veda*. Delhi: Atlantic Publishers.

22. Broek, R. V. *The Myth of The Phoenix accourding to Classical adn Early Christian Traditions*. BRILL.

23. Browne, E. G. (2011). *Arabian Medicine: The FitzPatrick Lectures Delivered at the College of Physicians in November 1919 and November 1920*. Cambridge University Press.

24. Buchbauer, K. H. (2015). *Handbook of Essential Oils: Science, Technology, and Applications, Second Edition*. CRC Press.

25. Charlesworth, J. H. (2010). *The Old Testament Pseudepigrapha: Apocalyptic literature and testaments*. Hendrickson Publishers.

26. Charran, S. R. *Sexual Death*. Lulu.com.

27. Chauhan, R. S., & Nautiyal, M. C. (2007, 12). *Seed germination and seed storage behaviour of Nardostachys jatamansi DC., an endangered medicinal herb of high-altitude Himalaya*. Retrieved 02 24, 2016, from Current Science:

http://connection.ebscohost.com/c/articles/25612546
/seed-germination-seed-storage-behaviour-
nardostachys-jatamansi-dc-endangered-medicinal-
herb-high-altitude-himalaya

28. Chauliac, G. D. (2007). *Commentary.* BRILL.

29. Clark, T. (1845). *Egypt and the Books of Moses: Or the Books of Egypt, with an Appendix.* T. Clark.

30. Culpepper, N. (2006). *Culpeper's Complete Herbal & English Physician.* Applewood Books.

31. Dhingra, D., & Goyal, P. K. (2008, 04). *Inhibition of MAO and GABA: Probable mechanisms for antidepressant-like activity of Nardostachys jatamansi DC. in mice.* Retrieved 03 01, 2016, from Niscar Online Articles Repository: http://nopr.niscair.res.in/handle/123456789/4455

32. Dispenza, J. (2010, 09 27). *Death and Rebirth: The Phoenix.* Retrieved 02 07, 2016, from Lifepath: http://www.lifepathretreats.com/death-and-rebirth-the-Phoenix

33. Dixit VP, J. P. (1988). *Hypolipidaemic effects of Curcuma longa L and Nardostachys jatamansi, DC in triton-induced*

hyperlipidaemic rats. Retrieved 03 01, 2016, from Europe PMC: http://europepmc.org/abstract/med/3215683

34. Duncan, A. *The Edinburgh New Dispensatory*. 1830: Bell & Bradfute.

35. E. Toolika, N. P. (2015, 03). *A comparative clinical study on the effect of Tagara (Valeriana wallichii DC.) and Jatamansi (Nardostachys jatamansi DC.) in the management of Anidra (primary insomnia)*. Retrieved 02 01, 2016, from Pubmed: http://www.ncbi.nlm.nih.gov/pmc/articles/PMC4687 238/

36. Edward Smedley, H. J. (1845). *Encyclopædia Metropolitana; Or, Universal Dictionary of Knowledge*. B Fellowes.

37. Efraim Lev, L. C. (2012). *Medical Prescriptions in the Cambridge Genizah Collections*. BRILL.

38. Efrayim Lev, Z. '. (2008). *Practical Materia Medica of the Medieval Eastern Mediterranean According to the Cairo Genizah*. BRILL.

39. Egan, H. D. (1991). *An Anthology of Christian Mysticism*. Liturgical Press.

40. Emmerlich, A. C. *The Dororous Passion of Our Lord Jesus Christ.* http://www.catholicplanet.com/ebooks/Dolorous-Passion.pdf.

41. Faas, P. (2013). *Around The Roman Table.* Pamn McMillian.

42. *Flight of The Phoenix - Image of Rebirth.* (n.d.). Retrieved 02 07, 2016, from Terrapsych: http://www.terrapsych.com/Phoenix.html

43. Forbes, R. J. (1955). *Studies in Ancient Technology, Volume 1.* E J Brill.

44. Gill, J. (1768). *An Exposition of the Book of Solomon's Song* . London: George Keith, Grace Street.

45. GI-SANG BAE, 1. K.-C.-J.-J.-J. (2012, 09). *Nardostachys jatamansi inhibits severe acute pancreatitis via mitogen-activated protein kinases.* Retrieved 02 01, 2016, from Pubmed: http://www.ncbi.nlm.nih.gov/pmc/articles/PMC3503632/

46. Gloria Karkada1, K. S. (2012). *Nardostachys jatamansi extract prevents chronic restraint stress-induced learning*

and memory deficits in a radial arm maze task. Retrieved 03 01, 2016, from Journal of Natural Science, Biology and Medicine: http://jnsbm.org/article.asp?issn=0976-9668;year=2012;volume=3;issue=2;spage=125;epage=132;aulast=Karkada

47. Granville, A. B. (1836). *The Sunbul.*

48. Gray, S. F. *Gray's Supplement to the Pharmacopoeia: Being a Concise But Comprehensive Dispensatory and Manual of Facts and Formulae, for the Chemist and Druggist and Medical Practitioner.* 1848: Longman and Company; & Highley, Simpkin and Company; John Churchill; Henry Bohn; and Henry Renshaw,.

49. Gryphon, L. (n.d.). *Phoenix.* Retrieved 02 11, 2016, from Mythical Realm: http://mythicalrealm.com/creatures/Phoenix.html

50. Halpern, M. (2016). *Majja Dhatu: A closer look at the nervous system from the ayurvedic perspective .* Retrieved 02 01, 2016, from California College of Ayurveda: http://www.ayurvedacollege.com/articles/drhalpern/Majja%20Dhatu

51. Hatchett, C. (1836). *On the spikenard of the ancients (by C. Hatchett).*

52. Himalaya Wellness. (n.d.). *Musk Root* . Retrieved 14 01, 2016, from Himalaya Wellness: http://www.himalayawellness.com/herbalmonograph/musk-root.htm

53. Holland, E. (2005). *Holland's Grimoire of Magickal Correspondences: A Ritual Handbook*. New Page Books.

54. Hone, W. (1820). *The Apocryphal New Testament*.

55. Horace, C. A. (1844). *The works of Horace: with English notes, critical and explanatory*. Harper and Brothers .

56. Hosking, R. (2005). *Authenticity in the Kitchen:*. Oxford: Proceedings of the Oxford Symposium on Food and Cookery.

57. *How Food Becomes Your Body*. (2014). Retrieved 02 16, 2016, from Eat Tast Heal: http://www.eattasteheal.com/ayurveda101/ETH_Tissues.htm

58. Hunt, P. (2008). *Poetry in the Song of Songs: A Literary Analysis*. Peter Lang.

59. Huntingford, G. W. (2010). *The Periplus of the Erythraean Sea, Volume 2, Part 4, Issue 151*. Hakluyt Societ.

60. Jackson, R. B. (2002). *At Empire's Edge: Exploring Rome's Egyptian Frontier.* Yale University Press.

61. Jenks, W. (1836). *The Comprehensive Commentary on the Holy Bible: Matt.-John.* Fessenden and Company.

62. John H. Wiersema, B. L. (2013). *World Economic Plants: A Standard Reference, Second Edition.* CRC Press.

63. John Shore, W. J. (1815). *Memoirs of the Life, Writings and Correspondence of Sir William Jones.* Hatchard.

64. Jones, S. W. (1807). *The Works of Sir William Jones: With the Life of the Author by Lord Teignmouth ..., Volume 5.* John Stockdale, Piccadilly; and John Walker, Paternoster-Row.

65. Karkada G1, S. K. (2012, 07). *Nardostachys jatamansi extract prevents chronic restraint stress-induced learning and memory deficits in a radial arm maze task.* Retrieved 03 01, 2016, from Pubmed: http://www.ncbi.nlm.nih.gov/pubmed/23225973

66. Kumar, R. (2010). *Essays on Indian Economy.* Discovery Publishing House.

67. Lang, A. (2013). *Red Book of Animal Stories.* Tuttle Publishing.

68. *Legends.* (n.d.). Retrieved 02 07, 2016, from Phoenix Arises: http://www.Phoenixarises.com/Phoenix/legends/legends.htm

69. Lyle N1, C. S. (2012, 12). *Nardostachys jatamansi protects against cold restraint stress induced central monoaminergic and oxidative changes in rats.* Retrieved 03 01, 2016, from Pubmed: http://www.ncbi.nlm.nih.gov/pubmed/229034704

70. Lyle, N., Bhattacharyya, D., Sur, T. K., Munshi, S., Paul, S., Chatterjee, S., et al. (2009, 02). *Stress modulating antioxidant effect of Nardostachys jatamansi.* Retrieved 03 01, 2016, from Niscar Online Articles Repository: http://nopr.niscair.res.in/handle/123456789/3323

71. M, J. V., M., T. R., K.J., K., & S., K. S. (2009). *Herbal Axiolyte: Nardostachys jatamansi.* Retrieved 02 24, 2016, from Journal of Pharmacy Research: http://www.cabdirect.org/abstracts/20103127134.html

72. Mackenzie, D. A. *Indian Myth and Legend (Illustrations).* The Gresham Publishing Company Limited.

73. Madan Mohan Pandey, A. K. (2013, 03). *An Important Indian Traditional Drug of Ayurveda Jatamansi and Its Substitute Bhootkeshi: Chemical Profiling and Antioxidant Activity.* Retrieved 07 01, 2016, from pUBMED: http://www.ncbi.nlm.nih.gov/pmc/articles/PMC3618914/

74. Madhulika Bhagat1*, 2. P.-I.-I. (2013, 11 25). *In vitro and In vivo Biological Activities of Nardostachys Jatamansi Roots.* Retrieved 02 24, 2016, from Medicinal and Aromatic Plants: http://www.omicsgroup.org/journals/in-vitro-and-in-vivo-biological-activities-of-nardostachys-jatamansi-roots.pdf-2167-0412.1000142.php?aid=21950

75. Mahmoud Etebari, B. Z.-D. (2012, 08). *Evaluation of DNA damage of hydro-alcoholic and aqueous extract of Echium amoenum and Nardostachys jatamansi.* Retrieved 02 01, 2016, from Pubmed: http://www.ncbi.nlm.nih.gov/pmc/articles/PMC3687887/

76. Maire, B. (2014). *'Greek' and 'Roman' in Latin Medical Texts: Studies in Cultural Change and Exchange in Ancient Medicine.* BRILL.

77. *Majja Dhattu*. (2013, 10 26). Retrieved 03 01, 2016, from Ayurveda and Yoga: https://ayurvedayogi.wordpress.com/2013/10/26/majja-dhatu-the-bone-marrow-tissue/

78. Malan, S. C. (2005). *The Book Of Adam And Eve*. Book Tree.

79. Margarita Gleba, J. P.-S. (2013). *Making Textiles in pre-Roman and Roman Times: People, Places, Identities*. Oxbow Books.

80. *Meaning Of The Phoenix*. (n.d.). Retrieved 02 11, 2016, from Signology.com: http://www.signology.org/bird-symbol/Phoenix-symbol.htm

81. MISHRA, D., V., C. R., & C., T. S. (1995). *The fungitoxic effect of the essential oil of the herb Nardostachys jatamansi DC*. Retrieved 03 01, 2016, from Refdoc.fr: http://cat.inist.fr/?aModele=afficheN&cpsidt=3529058

82. Mones Abu-Asab, P. H. (2013). *Avicenna's Medicine: A New Translation of the 11th-Century Canon with Practical Applications for Integrative Health Care*. Inner Traditions / Bear & Co,.

83. Monro, J. M. (1995). *Spikenard and Saffron: The Imagery of the Song of Songs.* Continnuum-3PL .

84. Muzamil Ahmada, ,. 1. (2006, 01). *Attenuation by Nardostachys jatamansi of 6-hydroxydopamine-induced parkinsonism in rats: behavioral, neurochemical, and immunohistochemical studies.* Retrieved 03 01, 2016, from Science   Direct: http://www.sciencedirect.com/science/article/pii/S0 091305706000098

85. MVIRDC World Trade Centre. (2002). *Export potential of herbal and ayurvedic drugs.* Bombay: The Centre with Quest Publications.

86. *Nardostachys jatamansi* . (2014-2015). Retrieved 03 02, 2016, from The IUCN Red List of Threatened Species(tm): http://www.iucnredlist.org/details/50126627/0

87. Nazmun Lylea, A. G. (2009, 09). *The role of antioxidant properties of Nardostachys jatamansi in alleviation of the symptoms of the chronic fatigue syndrome.* Retrieved 03 01, 2016,   from   Science   Direct: http://www.sciencedirect.com/science/article/pii/S0 166432809002216

88. Nutton, V. (2013). *Ancient Medicine*. Routledge.

89. *Oils and Herbs for Capricorn*. (n.d.). Retrieved 02 14, 2016, from The Untamed Alchemist : http://theuntamedalchemist.com/tag/spikenard/

90. P. N. Ravindran, K. N.-B. (2005). *Cinnamon and Cassia: The Genus Cinnamomum*. CRC Press.

91. Parle, H. J. (2006, 03). *Nardostachys jatamansi Improves Learning and Memory in Mice*. Retrieved 03 01, 2016, from Mary Licbert: http://online.liebertpub.com/doi/abs/10.1089/jmf.2006.9.113

92. Parr, B. (1809). *The London Medical Dictionary, Including Under Distinct Heads Every Branch of Medicine*. London .

93. Peregrine Horden, S. K. (2014). *A Companion to Mediterranean History*. John Wiley and Sons.

94. Pereira, J. (2013). *The Elements of Materia Medica and Therapeutics, Part 2*. Cambridge University Press,.

95. *Phoenix*. (n.d.). Retrieved 02 11, 2016, from New World Encyclopaedia: http://www.newworldencyclopedia.org/entry/Phoenix_(mythology)

96. *Phoenix*. (n.d.). Retrieved 02 11, 2016, from Bestiary: http://bestiary.ca/beasts/beast149.htm

97. *Phoenix*. (n.d.). Retrieved 02 11, 2016, from Crystalink: http://www.crystalinks.com/Phoenix.html

98. *Phoenix*. (2014). Retrieved 02 11, 2016, from Egyptian Myths: http://www.egyptianmyths.net/Phoenix.htm

99. Plants for The Future. (n.d.). *Nardostachys grandiflora*. Retrieved 02 02, 2016, from http://www.pfaf.org/user/Plant.aspx?LatinName=Nardostachys+grandiflora

100.   Prioreschi, P. (1966). *A History of Medicine: Roman medicine*. Horatius Press.

101.   Rajinder K. Gupta, J. D. (2014). *A Review on Spikenard (Nardostachysjatamansi DC.)- An 'Endangered' Essential Herb of India*. Retrieved 03 02, 2016, from International Journal of Pharmaceutical Chemistry: http://www.ssjournals.com/index.php/ijpc/article/view/1286

102.   Rawlinson, G. (2004). *The Seven Great Monarchies of the Ancient Eastern World, Or: Media; Babylonia; Persia*. Gorgias Press.

103.   Rawlinson, H. G. (1916). *Intercourse Between India and the Western World: From the Earliest Times of* . Asian Educational Services,India.

104.   Redwood, T. (1857). *A supplement to the pharmacopoia*. Longman.

105.   Rees, A. (1819). *The Cyclopaedia*. Longman, Hurst,.

106.   Regents' Professor of Egyptian Archaeology Richard H Wilkinson, K. R. (2016). *The Oxford Handbook To The Valley Of the Kings*. Oxford University Press.

107.   Rhind, J. P. (2013). *Fragrance and Wellbeing: Plant Aromatics and Their Influence on the Psyche*. Singing Dragon.

108.   Rimmel, E. (1865). *The Book of Perfumes*. Chapman & Hall,.

109.   Rosenmüller, E. F. (1836). *The Biblical Geography of Central Asia:*. Thomas Clark.

110.   Rosner, F. (2000). *Encyclopedia of Medicine in the Bible and the Talmud*. Jason Aronson.

111.   Royle, J. F. (1839). *Illustrations of the botany and other branches of the natural history of the the Himalayan mountains (etc.).* Allen.

112.   Rupali A. Patil, Y. A. (2012, 05). *Reversal of reserpine-induced orofacial dyskinesia and catalepsy by Nardostachys jatamansi.* Retrieved 03 01, 2016, from Pubmed: http://www.ncbi.nlm.nih.gov/pmc/articles/PMC3371456/

113.   Sami Khalaf Hamarneh, G. A. (1963). *A Pharmaceutical View of Abulcasis Al-Zahrāwī in Moorish Spain.* BRILL.

114.   Sandeep PM1, B. T. (2015, 08). *Anti-Androgenic Activity of Nardostachys jatamansi DC and Tribulus terrestris L. and Their Beneficial Effects on Polycystic Ovary Syndrome-Induced Rat Models.* Retrieved 02 01, 2016, from   Pubmed: http://www.ncbi.nlm.nih.gov/pubmed/25919204

115.   Sawer, J. C. (1894). *Odorographia a natural history of raw materials and drugs used in the perfume industry intended to serve growers manufacturers and consumers.* Рипол Классик.

116.   Schoff, W. (1923). Nard. *Journal of the American Oriental Society* , pp. Vol. 43 (1923), pp. 216-228.

117.   Shakir Alia, K. A. (2000, 08). *Nardostachys jatamansi protects against liver damage induced by thioacetamide in rats.* Retrieved 03 01, 2016, from Science Direct: http://www.sciencedirect.com/science/article/pii/S0 378874199001531

118.   Shin JY1, B. G. (2015, 12 29). *Anti-inflammatory effect of desoxo-narchinol-A isolated from Nardostachys jatamansi against lipopolysaccharide.* Retrieved 03 01, 2016, from Pubmed: http://www.ncbi.nlm.nih.gov/pubmed/26371857

119.   Simpson, S. J. (1872). *Archaeological Essays: On leprosy and leper hospitals in Scotland and England.* Edmonston and Douglas,.

120.   Sofiyan Salim, M. A. (2003, 01). *Protective effect of Nardostachys jatamansi in rat cerebral ischemia.* Retrieved 03 01, 2016, from Science Direct: http://www.sciencedirect.com/science/article/pii/S0 091305702010304

121.   *Spikenard*. (n.d.). Retrieved 25 02, 2016, from Herb   world: http://www.herbworld.com/learningherbs/SPIKENA RD.pdf

122.   *Spikenard*. (n.d.). Retrieved 20 25, 2016, from Everything   explained: http://everything.explained.today/Spikenard/

123.   *Spikenard*. (n.d.). Retrieved 02 25, 2016, from Aromasana: http://www.aromasana.com/SPIKENARD.pdf

124.   *Spikenard*. (n.d.). Retrieved 02 02, 2016, from http://www.jonnsaromatherapy.com/eoS-Z.html#Spikenard

125.   *Spikenard*. (2016). Retrieved 02 25, 2502, from Wikepedia: https://en.wikipedia.org/wiki/Spikenard

126.   *Spikenard, Or Nard*. (n.d.). Retrieved 02 21, 2016, from   Library   Index: http://www.libraryindex.com/encyclopedia/pages/c pxlbml7z1/spikenard-nard-root-ointment.html

127.   *Symbolic Meaning of The Phoenix*. (n.d.). Retrieved 02   11,   2016,   from   Whats-Your-Sign:

http://www.whats-your-sign.com/symbolic-meaning-of-the-Phoenix.html

128.   Tanishka. (2014). *Creating Sacred Union in Partnerships.* Star of Ishtar Publishing .

129.   Taylor, C. (1814). *Scripture illustrated by means of natural Science: in botany, geology and Geogrpahy.* Tylor.

130.   *The Asiatic Journal and Monthly Miscellany,.* (1835). Wm. H. Allen & Company.

131.   Tilton, H. (2003). *The Quest for the Phoenix: Spiritual Alchemy and Rosicrucianism in the Workin the Work of Count Michael Maier (1569-1622).* Walter de Gruyter.

132.   Totelin, L. M. (2009). *Hippocratic Recipes: Oral and Written Transmission of Pharmacological knowledge in Fifth and Forth Century Greece.* BRILL.

133.   Venkateswara Rao Gottumukkala, T. A. (2011, 06). *Phytochemical investigation and hair growth studies on the rhizomes of Nardostachys jatamansi DC.* Retrieved 02 24, 2016, from Pubmed: http://www.ncbi.nlm.nih.gov/pmc/articles/PMC3113 354/

134.   Vidya S. Raoa, ,. ,. (2005, Dec). *Anticonvulsant and neurotoxicity profile of Nardostachys jatamansi in rats.* Retrieved 03 01, 2016, from Science Direct: http://www.sciencedirect.com/science/article/pii/S0 37887410500423X

135.   Weberling, F. (1975, August). On The Systemics of Jatamansi. *International Association for Plant Taxonomy (IAPT)* , pp. 443-452.

136.   William Milburn, T. T. (1825). *East India Trader's Complete Guide.* Kingsbury, Parbury, and Allen,.

137.   Winner, D. (2012). *Al Dente: Madness, Beauty and the Food of Rome.* Simon and Schuster.

138.   Worwood, V. A. (2013). *The Fragrant Heavens.* Transworld Digital.

Bibliography

- Healing the Spirit- Gabriel Mojay
- The World of Aromatherapy - Jeanne Rose
- Kurt Schnaubelt – The Healing Intelligence of Essential Oils
- Essential Oil Safety Tisserand and Young 2013

- Sacred Luxuries – Dr Lise Manniche - Sacred Luxuries. Fragrance, Aromatherapy, and Cosmetics in Ancient Egypt.
- Sexual Secrets: The Alchemy of Ecstasy: Penny Slinger and Nik Douglas

Made in the USA
San Bernardino, CA
14 October 2016